DOCTOR HOMOLA'S
NATURAL HEALTH REMEDIES

Books by Samuel Homola, D.C.

Bonesetting, Chiropractic, and Cultism
Backache: Home Treatment and Prevention
A Chiropractor's Treasury of Health Secrets
(Los Secretos de la Salud Tratamientos Quiropracticos)
Muscle Training for Athletes
Secrets of Naturally Youthful Health and Vitality

DOCTOR HOMOLA'S
NATURAL HEALTH REMEDIES

Samuel Homola, D.C.

Foreword by
Jonathan Forman, B.A., M.D., F.A.C.A., F.I.C.A.N.

Parker Publishing Company, Inc. West Nyack, N.Y.

Dedicated to my father, the late Dr. Joseph Homola.

Library of Congress Cataloging in Publication Data

Homola, Samuel.
    Doctor Homola's natural health remedies.

    1. Chiropractic. I. Title. [DNLM: 1. Naturo-
pathy. WB960 H768d 1973]
RZ241.H65   615'.535   73-7552
ISBN 0-13-216945-2

Foreword by a Doctor of Medicine

This book by a Doctor of Chiropractic deals with natural self-help remedies that should be useful to persons of all ages. It is now generally well known that good health depends upon good nutrition and good living habits. It is also well known that there are a multitude of ailments that are best cared for with simple, drugless remedies that are within the reach of everyone. Natural remedies and natural foods build good health, and they help to prevent diseases and illnesses that shorten life.

The programs outlined in this book are based on natural laws that form a common denominator for all healing methods, and they represent a sincere effort to help people who want to help themselves. No one can dispute the value of natural foods, moist heat, and other natural techniques that should be a part of every individual's effort to ease his aches and pains and prolong his life.

You are personally responsible for your health and the care of your body. You must read and study books such as this, if you are to be knowledgeable enough to help yourself and protect your health. You must be broad-minded in your search for effective ways to care for your body. In the final analysis, you alone must make the final judgement of the effectiveness of remedies and measures that affect your health.

This book by Samuel Homola describes many safe, simple natural remedies and health-building measures that could be recommended by any practitioner who is sincerely concerned about helping others. I therefore recommend this book for all those who are searching for drugless remedies that are designed to build health as well as relieve suffering.

Jonathan Forman, B.A., M.D., F.A.C.A.,
F.I.C.A.N.

What This Book Can Do For You

The average family spends several hundred dollars and upwards each year on medical bills. Much of this may be spent for simple, minor ailments that could be handled successfully at home without professional care.

Unfortunately, few doctors have the time to tell their patients how to help themselves. With illness so rampant and doctors so overworked, only "serious" disorders receive adequate attention in the average doctor's office. The truth is, however, that many "minor" disorders can develop into serious diseases when they are neglected. And if they aren't handled with natural healing methods that stimulate the healing powers of the body, they may never be completely cured.

There are millions of people who are suffering from minor and chronic ailments that would respond immediately to properly applied natural remedies. Few of these people are aware of the fact that their suffering could be relieved at home. What about you? Are you suffering from some nagging ailment that makes your life miserable? Your body has a remarkable capacity to heal itself when it is helped along by natural healing methods.

In this book, I have outlined basic home-treatment methods for a great variety of common and not-so-common ailments, and I show you how to help your body heal itself naturally. For less than the price of one office call, you can acquire more health guidance from this book than a doctor could give you in a hundred office calls—and the book is yours to keep for the rest of your life. Regular use of this book will cut down your health expenses, as well as tell you exactly what to do to help yourself and relieve your suffering. *You* can care for many of your ailments as effectively as the most expensive specialist. You don't have to

6

run to an overworked doctor's office every time you have a muscle spasm, a cold, or a headache.

Remember that *only nature heals*. Any treatment that may be of value to you as a home remedy must aid nature without harming your body. So don't confuse natural healing methods with patent medicines that do nothing but choke off symptoms. Some drugs actually *delay* healing by interfering with the internal processes of the body. Natural remedies improve body functions as a whole, thus improving your health and prolonging your life.

With this book, you'll have a handy and easy-to-read guide to reliable and effective natural remedies that can be used by every member of your family. You'll learn how to handle hundreds of ailments with tried and proven natural healing methods that have produced prompt results for a great many people. The home remedies in this book combine healing science with "folk medicine" and "health secrets" in a self-help program that I am confident will work as well for you as it does for me and my patients.

There are several special features for your health benefit in this book. As a practicing chiropractor, I'm able to bring you many new methods of treatment that have not been described, to the best of my knowledge, in books written for laymen. A new spinal manipulation technique, for example, that can be used safely at home by anyone, will do wonders in relieving aches and pains that do not respond to conventional treatment methods. Also, my work in training and treating athletes enables me to bring you many new and effective treatment methods that have been designed to produce rapid and lasting results.

This is *not* one of those books that dwells only on nutrition, body mechanics, or some other specialized method of healing. This book tells you how to use *all* the natural remedies and healing methods, and how to apply them to *all* the ailments that can be cared for at home.

However, if I had to give the methods in this book one all-encompassing name, I would call them "Naturomatic Healing," because the whole system of natural healing which I describe seems to work automatically to help your body heal itself, and restore its natural health balance. Thus, each and every technique mentioned in the book might be considered part of the Naturomatic Healing Method.

Samuel Homola, D.C.

Contents

Hardened arteries cause many diseases . How to relieve the symptoms of Atherosclerosis with dietary methods . How you benefit from eating low-fat, protein foods . Eat more fruits and vegetables . Cut out refined carbohydrates . Increase your intake of unsaturated fat . Make sure you get adequate Vitamin F . How lecithin helps melt the hard fat in your arteries . How certain B vitamins help control blood fat . Vitamin E heals your heart and helps your arteries . Paul E's success with Vitamin E . A special diet and a herbal drink for heart pain . A special bath to relax your heart patients . How to handle leg pain caused by hardened arteries . How to walk away the pain of hardened arteries before it's "too late" . How one man regained his ability to walk long distances . A bedroom program for improving circulation in legs that have been crippled by hardened arteries . How to do the Buerger bed exercises . How to aid circulation with wooden blocks and alcohol . The proper way to use heat to improve circulation . How to lower your blood pressure with natural methods . How Josephine coped with her high blood pressure . Reduce the sugar and animal fat in your diet for more flexible arteries . Why you should restrict your intake of salt to reduce water pressure . Salt substitutes . Eat as much fresh fruit as possible for special vitamins and   minerals . Reduce your body weight to get rid of parasitic blood vessels . A rice diet will reduce blood pressure . Open up your blood vessels with garlic . How John H. took the lid off his emotional stress . How to cope with low blood pressure and dizzy spells . A special diet for low blood pressure . How to aid

1. **How to Extend Your Life with Naturomatic Healing of Heart and Blood Vessel Diseases** *(cont.)*

    circulation in varicose veins . How to elevate your legs to drain swollen veins . How to use a compression bandage to prevent filling of enlarged veins . How to pump blood with leg muscles and water pressure . How to use a "Gelatin Boot" for speedy healing of a varicose ulcer . How to use a simple rubber-and-bandage wrapping for small ulcers . A contrast bath will benefit varicose ulcers . How to relieve the agony of phlebitis

    How to relieve the symptoms of emphysema . The match test for emphysema . How to moisturize the air you breathe . How to empty your bronchial tubes with postural drainage . How to combine breathing and walking to relieve breathlessness . How to empty your lungs with positive pressure breathing . A better diet for faster healing of lungs . Hints for victims of asthma, hay fever, and other allergies . Remove irritating elements from the air you breathe . Check your diet for food allergies . How to correct nutritional deficiencies . How to control allergies by controlling your blood sugar . How to relieve asthma by controlling your emotions . You can exhale easier with a bottle of water . How to take effective action against the common cold . Increase your intake of Vitamin C . Bathe your throat with acid vapor . Kill cold germs with garlic and onion . Control the temperature and humidity of your home . General measures to relieve a clogged or dry nose and other symptoms . How to soothe a sore throat and cope with tonsillitis . How to relieve a sore throat with hot drinks and seaweed lemonade . How to use fomentations for a sore throat . An overnight heating compress for sore throat . How to use hot packs and cold packs to relieve tonsillitis . How to get quick relief for inflammation of the nose, throat, sinuses, and chest . How to use medicated steam for aggravating coughs . How to use cold packs and hot foot baths to relieve acute sinusitis . How to unclog your nose and sinuses with irrigation . How onion can clean your nose . How to use a penetrating mustard plaster for chest soreness . How to relieve lung congestion caused by respiratory infection . How to ease the stabbing pain of pleurisy . How Billy J. handled his pleurisy attack . How to reduce a fever . How to care for diaphragmatic hernia . How to control nervous breathing and hiccups . How to eliminate the causes of bad breath . Clean out your mouth . Brush your tongue . Balance the bacterial content of your intestinal tract

8. **Tested Naturomatic Healing Methods for Headache,
   Constipation and Hemorrhoids** *(cont.)*

*visit the toilet regularly . Step 3: take an enema when necessary .
Step 4: eat moisture-retaining foods . A special non-irritating bulk
diet . Carbohydrates, constipation, and cancer . How to soothe the
burning, itching pain of hemorrhoids . Protect hemorrhoids with
a proper diet . How to lubricate your hemorrhoids with olive oil .
How to make an anal steam bath . How to replace protruding
internal hemorrhoids . How to soothe the painful agony of an anal
fissure . How to ease an "itching bottom"*

*A simple home-care program for peptic ulcer . How to relieve pain
and promote healing of stomach ulcers by eating special foods .
Drink more milk and go easy on alkalizers . Special advice for victims
of obesity and hardened arteries . How to make corn-oil milk . Milk
substitutes for allergy victims . How to mix an effective household
alkalizer . How to make potato and cabbage alkalizers . How to
relieve stomach pain with an ice bag . How to eat so that a stomach
ulcer can heal itself . How to make ulcer-healing cream soups . How
to relieve constipation caused by an ulcer diet . How to cure ulcers
by relieving emotional stress . How to relieve indigestion caused by
stomach acid deficiency . How to improve your digestion with acids
and enzymes . Hints for relieving ordinary indigestion . Don't rush
your meals! Quit smoking before dinner—and go easy on coffee .
Eliminate grease and fat—and eat fresh, natural foods . Get your
teeth in shape . Go easy on gas-forming foods—and declare war on
gas-forming bacteria . How to take a special enema to relieve gas
pressure . How to relieve abdominal pain with hot packs . Measures
for coping with simple diarrhea . Clean your intestine with a 24-hour
fast . Check diarrhea with buttermilk and bananas . How to correct
dehydration caused by diarrhea . Warning: milk causes diarrhea in
some people . How to cope with colitis and diverticulitis . Colitis,
food, and mind power . How to handle an inflamed, constipated
colon . The cause and cure of diverticulitis . How to eat to relieve
diverticulitis*

*How to stop the progress of pyorrhea and other gum diseases . How
to recognize the early warning signs of gum disease . Home care for
your teeth and gums . How to improve the health of your teeth and*

15. **Miscellaneous Naturomatic Remedies for a Variety of**
Injuries and Ailments *(cont.)*

*How to stop nausea . How to ease gas pains . How to stop hiccups .
What to do about fever blisters . Hints on the care of shingles . How
to treat rosacea . How to eliminate hives . How to restore color to
gray hair . How to crase skin wrinkles . How to ease the swelling of a
black eye . How to get a cinder out of your eye . How to clean out
your ears . How to strengthen a ruptured abdomen . How to reduce
nervous tremors . How to wrap stubbed toes and fingers . How to
lose excess body fat . First aid for acid and alkali burns . First aid for
spinal fractures . Nutritional therapy for all diseases*

1

How to Extend Your Life with Naturomatic Healing of Heart and Blood Vessel Diseases

Each year more than 600,000 Americans die from heart attacks! The way of life of the average American practically guarantees the development of arterial disease that will cause the heart to fail in the prime of life—but that doesn't have to happen to *you*. You'll learn in this chapter how to use simple, natural methods to correct such disorders as atherosclerosis, high blood pressure, and overweight—and the remedies you use will help to extend your life with a youthfully healthier heart.

Jack B. was only 50 years of age when he began to suffer from fatigue, high blood pressure, chest pain, leg ache, and ringing in his ears. When I learned that he had a high blood fat with hardening of the arteries, I recommended that he follow the suggestions outlined in this chapter. "What's the use?" he argued. "My father and my brother died of heart attacks before they were 60 years old. My last doctor told me that I have probably inherited arterial disease. So why torture myself with a weird diet?"

Jack B., like many people who die young, had *not* inherited a tendency toward heart disease. He was simply eating the same way his father and his grandfather had eaten. Each generation had passed their bad eating habits to the next generation. When I convinced Jack B. that such cooking practices as adding sugar and bacon grease to vegetables could cause cardiovascular disease, he reluctantly agreed to follow my advice. Several months later, his blood fat was nearly normal and most of his symptoms had disappeared. "I never would have believed it, Doctor," he said with amazement. "I was resigned to die young with all my aches and pains. But now I feel great. My new goal in life is to live to be a hundred years old!"

Hardened Arteries Cause Many Diseases

When hardened arteries interfere with the circulation of blood, it's not just the heart that's affected. Many things can go wrong in other portions of the body. Poor circulation around the brain, for example, may cause dizziness, loss of memory, and inability to think. A disturbance in the inner ear may cause vertigo and tinnitus, or "ringing in the ears." Stroke, phlebitis, Buerger's disease, and other circulatory diseases may result from the formation of clots in spastic blood vessels. Oxygen deficiency in the legs may make it impossible to walk more than a few steps without excruciating cramps or leg pain. Exertion results in shortness of breath and chest pain (angina pectoris). Blood pressure rises, and the inability of the blood vessels to expand with each heart beat causes thumping pressures that may damage important organs. Blurred vision may occur from hardening of retinal arteries. Physical changes lead to premature aging, and so on. If you're suffering from hardened or clogged arteries (also called arteriosclerosis or atherosclerosis), there's much that you can do to *reverse* the process and relieve the symptoms.

How to Relieve the Symptoms of Atherosclerosis with Dietary Methods

Cholesterol and hard fat are the biggest offenders in hardened or clogged arteries. Cholesterol isn't a fat, but it's usually associated with the hard or saturated fat in foods of animal origin. This means that you can cut down on both cholesterol and saturated fat simply by reducing your intake of animal fat.

How you benefit from eating
low-fat, protein foods

Get most of your animal protein from fish, chicken, *uncreamed* cottage cheese, and skim milk, all of which are low in saturated fat. When you do buy other types of meat, always select lean cuts, and then trim away all the visible fat before you begin cooking. All meats should be cooked over a slotted broiling pan so that the "invisible" fat can drop into a bottom pan for disposal. Don't use any form of animal fat (such as bacon grease or butter) in cooking. And try not to eat bakery products containing butter, lard, margarine, hydrogenated shortening, and other solid fats. Go easy on eating egg yolk and organ meats. Use only those milk products made from skim milk.

Eat more fruits and vegetables

Eat a variety of fresh fruits and vegetables every day. Fruits, such as apples, contain pectin and Vitamin C, which help to lower blood cholesterol.

Cut out refined carbohydrates

Completely eliminate all white-sugar and white-flour products from your diet. There is now considerable evidence to indicate that excessive use of refined carbohydrates—especially sugar— contributes greatly to the development of atherosclerosis. Even children who eat such foods show signs of arterial disease.

Increase your intake
of unsaturated fat

In order to make sure that the hard fat in your diet is kept in a liquid state so that it can circulate freely in your arteries, you should increase your intake of *soft or unsaturated vegetable fat.*

You can do this by using vegetable oil in your cooking and by eating seeds, nuts, avocados, and other "oily" fruits and vegetables.

Remember, however, that too much fat of any kind, saturated or unsaturated, will contribute extra calories. So try to *cut down on the total amount of fat in your diet so that you get only about 25 percent of your calories from fat, with two-thirds of them coming from vegetable sources.*

Make sure you get
adequate Vitamin F

Don't ever try to eliminate all the fat in your diet. Without the essential fatty acids (Vitamin F) supplied by vegetable oil, the cholesterol normally manufactured by your body cannot be used in the construction of healthy tissue. (When linoleic acid is supplied by vegetable oil, your body can manufacture the other fatty acids.)

If you don't think you eat enough vegetables, seeds, and nuts to supply the amount of unsaturated fat you need, you can add about two teaspoons of cold-pressed wheat germ oil, corn oil, or safflower oil to each meal. Just put the oil on salads, on toast, in vegetable juice, or on any food that proves to be palatable with oil. Fish liver oil is rich in unsaturated fat, and it will supply Vitamins A and D, which tend to be deficient in diets that are low in animal fat.

How lecithin helps melt the hard fat
in your arteries

Most natural foods that contain saturated fat also contain lecithin, a substance that keeps the fat soft and pliable. *Over-cooking or processing foods, however, destroys the lecithin,* leaving the saturated fat in concentrated form. If your diet doesn't consist entirely of natural foods, or if you must eat in restaurants frequently, it would be a good idea to supplement your diet with lecithin, especially if you're over forty years of age. Any drug store or health food store can supply you with pure lecithin in tablets, granules, or some other form. Soybeans and avocados are good sources of vegetable lecithin. With adequate lecithin in your diet, the cholesterol in your blood won't readily harden or stick to the walls of your arteries.

How certain B vitamins
help control blood fat

Choline, inositol, pyridoxin, and other B vitamins can be used by your body to manufacture lecithin. Processed foods, however, are usually deficient in B vitamins. If you aren't able to get bread, cereals, and other foods made from whole grains that haven't "been through the mill," you should add wheat germ or brewer's yeast to your diet. Both are exceptionally rich in B vitamins.

Vitamin E heals your heart
and helps your arteries

It's now known that Vitamin E conserves oxygen, dilates (opens up) blood vessels, and dissolves blood clots. It also keeps oxygen from destroying the essential fatty acids your body needs to dissolve the hard fat in your arteries—and the more unsaturated fat you have in your diet, the more Vitamin E you need.

You can get some additional Vitamin E as well as unsaturated fat from wheat germ, wheat germ oil, and all types of seeds and nuts. Back in the days before the use of refined foods became so common (and when death from coronary thrombosis was rare), the daily intake of Vitamin E probably averaged as much as 150 units per day. You may need as much as 300 units daily to overcome the fat that's already in your arteries. If you have any type of heart or arterial disease, you should try taking several hundred units of Vitamin E daily for awhile. Persons with high blood pressure, however, should be cautious about taking very large doses of Vitamin E, and get professional advice, since it tends to raise blood pressure by increasing the tone of the heart muscle. Begin with about 100 units daily and slowly increase the amount if no ill effects are observed.

Paul E's success with Vitamin E

A famous Canadian physician who has pioneered the use of Vitamin E in treating heart disease reports that use of this vitamin has restored many incapacitated heart patients to a normal and active life. He tells of one 65-year-old patient, Paul E., who developed congestive heart failure after two coronary occlusions. Paul was so near death that he had to gasp for breath and remain in a sitting position in bed. His abdomen was greatly distended with fluid, and his legs were greatly swollen from circulatory failure. Conventional medical care had failed to halt the progress of the disease. After only two weeks of treatment with Vitamin E, however, Paul E. was able to get out of bed. A few months later, he went back to work. Three years later, he built his doctor a cottage!

A Special Diet and a Herbal Drink for Heart Pain

Most heart pain occurs near the center of the chest and is described as a squeezing or crushing sensation—as if a vise were being clamped around the chest. The sensation will occasionally radiate down into the left arm or up into the neck. If the pain is caused by hardened or clogged arteries, it will usually disappear with rest. The pain will keep recurring, however, if something isn't done to flush out the arteries. A good low-fat diet that includes lecithin, vegetable oil, and plenty of Vitamin E (as in treating atherosclerosis), along with regular walking exercises may eventually afford complete relief.

Many practitioners of folk medicine maintain that an *infusion of hawthorn berries* helps the heart by dilating (opening up) the coronary arteries. Just put a tablespoonful of dried berries into a cup of boiling water and let them soak in a warm place for about 20 minutes. Then strain the infusion and squeeze the berries. You can sweeten the drink with honey and enrich it with Vitamin C by stirring in powdered rose hips. (These ingredients can usually be secured at a health food store.)

A Special Bath to Relax Your Heart and Normalize Your Blood Pressure

A slightly warm carbon dioxide bath is reported to be beneficial in relieving the workload on the heart by slowing the heart rate and dilating blood vessels. It will tend to *lower* high blood pressure and *raise* low blood pressure.

To make this highly beneficial bath, add four to eight pounds of salt to a tub containing about 40 gallons of water. Then add one-half pound of sodium bicarbonate and six to eight large tablets of sodium sulfate. A rubber sheet can be used to protect the bottom of the tub from the action of the carbon dioxide gas that's generated.

Lie quietly in the bubbly, tingling water for about ten minutes and let the carbon dioxide bubbles accumulate on your skin. Dilatation of the blood vessels in your skin will give it a pleasant glow.

The carbon dioxide bath is a favorite in health spas where heart trouble is treated. You can purchase the chemicals for this bath in any drug store.

Hints for Heart Patients

When you're suffering from any type of heart or blood vessel disease, you should not smoke cigarettes. The nicotine of tobacco is a vasoconstrictor, which means that it reduces blood flow by narrowing the blood vessels. The caffeine in coffee is also a vasoconstrictor. So is emotional stress. When all these factors are combined, spasm of the coronary arteries can result in a heart attack without the actual formation of a thrombus or clot.

Overeating reduces the flow of blood to the heart muscle. It's especially important that you avoid exerting yourself right after eating a large meal.

Exertion during exposure to extremely cold wind, as in shoveling snow or walking uphill against a wintry wind, may trigger heart pain by reflexly constricting the arteries around the heart. When you are forced to work in a freezing wind, cover your nose and mouth with a scarf (or simply wear a surgical mask) in order to warm the air you breathe.

How to Handle Leg Pain
Caused by Hardened Arteries

When the arteries of the legs harden, poor circulation deprives the calf muscles of adequate oxygen. This causes *intermittent claudication,* or leg pain that interferes with walking. The pain usually occurs after a few minutes of walking, disappears with rest, and then recurs when walking is resumed. In severe cases, the victim may find it impossible to walk more than a few steps before the pain begins.

How to walk away the pain
of hardened arteries
before it's "too late"

Most people who first begin to experience leg pain during walking will simply quit walking to *avoid* the pain. This is usually a mistake. If the calf muscles aren't exercised by regular walking, the circulation in the legs becomes increasingly deficient. This means that a person who previously felt leg pain only after walking a couple of blocks will soon begin to experience pain after walking a few steps. In many cases, the leg pain never would have developed in the first place if long walks had been part of the daily routine. Regular use of your legs will improve circulation and open new blood vessels in your calf muscles, so that your legs will have adequate blood flow even in the presence of hardened arteries.

Walk some every day. Stop when leg pain or muscle spasm becomes intolerable, rest until the pain subsides, and then resume walking. Whenever possible, walk on pavement rather than on grass or dirt.

How one man regained his ability
to walk long distances

A 60-year-old optician who couldn't walk more than half a block without stopping because of leg pain confessed that he had quit walking years before the pain started. When he took a Vitamin E supplement and forced himself to walk some every day, he was soon able to walk several blocks without much discomfort. "It sure is great," he said, "to be able to walk again."

No matter how much trouble you're having with your leg arteries, you can regain your ability to walk if you'll combine dietary remedies with regular leg exercise.

A Bedroom Program for Improving Circulation in Legs
That Have Been Crippled by Hardened Arteries

If the circulation in your legs is so poor that you cannot walk more than a few steps without pain, there are some special bedroom exercises that you can do to stimulate circulation and to help prevent tissue destruction or gangrene.

How to do the Buerger
bed exercises

Several times a day, sit on the edge of a bed, dangle your legs, and then flex your feet and ankles in all directions for about three minutes. Contraction of the calf muscles while the legs are hanging down will pump blood through the arteries without creating an "oxygen debt." Then lie down on the bed and lift each leg up and down several times to use gravity in emptying and filling the veins and arteries. If you like, you can prop each foot up on a padded stool for several seconds at a time, but you shouldn't hold your legs in an elevated position after they blanch or turn white. Remember that arterial blood in the legs flows best while the legs are in a lowered position.

Note: If you have leg pain caused by hardened arteries, you shouldn't sit in reclining chairs that lift your legs higher than your hips.

How to aid circulation
with wooden blocks and alcohol

You can assure an improved flow of blood through diseased leg arteries during the night by placing blocks of wood, for example, under the head posts of your bed. This will place your body on a slight incline so that gravity can aid the flow of arterial blood to the legs.

If leg pain occurs while you are lying in bed, sit on the side of the bed and bend your ankles in all directions—or get up and walk around. If that doesn't help, sip one or two ounces of whiskey or brandy. Alcohol is a vasodilator; that is, it improves circulation by dilating or widening blood vessels. In many cases, it is just as effective as drugs for relieving pain caused by spasm of the arteries.

Niacin, a B vitamin, available in health food stores, will also dilate blood vessels.*

Warning: If obvious color or temperature changes take place around your feet and ankles, or if leg pain persists unrelieved, see your doctor as soon as possible. Buerger's disease, thrombophlebitis, and other vascular diseases can lead to clots or spasms that can completely obstruct the flow of blood through the legs.

The proper way to use heat to improve circulation

You should never apply hot packs or a heating pad to an area of the body where the circulation of blood has been impaired. In addition to the danger of burns, which can lead to ulcers or gangrene because of poor healing, excessive heat may create symptoms of oxygen deficiency (pain) by stimulating metabolic activity in the muscles.

Use only mildly warm moist heat applications (or sponge with warm water) to stimulate impaired circulation in the legs—or simply cover the legs with woolen blankets. In severe cases of arterial disease, heat applied to the abdomen can be used safely to reflexly dilate the blood vessels in the legs.

How to Lower Your Blood Pressure with Natural Methods

Normal blood pressure is usually said to be "120 over 80," which represents the highest pressure generated by contraction of the heart and the lowest pressure between contractions. These pressures vary in different persons, depending upon age, weight, and other factors. Generally speaking, when the first (systolic) pressure is above 150, or when the second (diastolic) pressure is

---

*Niacinamide offers all the utritional effects of niacin but it does *not* flush the blood vessels.

above 90, high blood pressure or hypertension should be suspected. Too much pressure in your arteries can cause such symptoms as headache, dizziness, weakness, fatigue, nervousness, insomnia, palpitation, and shortness of breath. It can also lead to stroke, hemorrhage, kidney damage, or heart failure. Millions of Americans have high blood pressure, and half of them aren't even aware that they have this dangerous disease.

How Josephine coped with her high blood pressure

Josephine C. was 41 before she discovered that she had high blood pressure. "I've never been sick," she said, "so I have never had a medical checkup. Lately, however, I've been feeling tired and nervous, and I don't sleep well at night."

Recordings of Josephine's blood pressure revealed that she had a dangerously high pressure. Simple, natural home treatment restored her pressure to normal in less than three months. "I've quit using table salt," she said, "and I'm eating plenty of fresh fruit." In addition to a reduction in blood pressure, Josephine lost *15 pounds* of excess body weight. "I feel fine," she said gleefully, "and I sleep good *every* night."

Even if you don't have high blood pressure, you can keep your blood pressure normal—and benefit in many other ways—by observing *all* the recommendations outlined in this chapter.

Note: If your doctor tells you that your blood pressure is high, ask him to take it two or three times at fifteen-minute intervals. Chances are your pressure will drop considerably when you are more relaxed and not so nervous.

Reduce the sugar and animal fat in your diet for more flexible arteries

Since hardened arteries and excessive blood fat contribute to the development of high blood pressure, you should observe the dietary measures recommended at the beginning of this chapter for combating arteriosclerosis and atherosclerosis.

Why you should restrict your intake
of salt to reduce water pressure

Do not use table salt in your cooking or on your food—or at least not more than one gram every 24 hours. (One-sixteenth of an ounce is about a gram and a half.) If you don't perspire heavily each day, you can get all the salt you need from *natural* foods. Try to prepare your own foods, and select *fresh* foods whenever possible. Canned or processed foods may contain salt or sodium additives.

Remember that it's the *sodium* in salt that increases your blood pressure by *hardening* your arteries and forcing your tissues to hold an excessive amount of water. For this reason, you should also reduce your intake of products containing baking soda, sodium additives, or antacids containing sodium bicarbonate. Read the labels on packaged foods. If the food contains sodium in any form, don't buy it. Water that is used for drinking, especially water that has been "softened" artificially, is often rich in sodium. Ask your local water department for an analysis of the water you drink. If it's high in sodium, and you have high blood pressure, you may have to distill the water, or buy bottled "low sodium" water.

Salt substitutes

Make sure that your diet includes seafood at least once a week so that you won't have to depend upon iodized salt for your iodine. If you don't like seafood, try sprinkling dried, powdered kelp on some of your foods. (Kelp is a seaweed that is rich in iodine and other minerals.) Rather than use salt to season your foods, you can use onions, toasted sesame seeds, pepper, horse-radish, garlic, celery seeds, sage, and other tasty herbs and spices. If you must use salt, purchase *natural sea salt* from a health food store.

Eat as much fresh fruit as possible
for special vitamins and minerals

No matter what type of diet you're on, plenty of fresh fruit should be helpful in reducing blood pressure. Remember that the pectin found in the pulp of fruit helps to prevent hardening of the arteries. So be sure to eat the whole fruit rather than squeeze it for juice. Fruits are also rich in potassium, which counteracts excessive sodium in your system. And they contain Vitamin C and Vitamin P (rutin and bioflavonoids), which help to strengthen blood vessels as well as lower blood pressure.

Reduce your body weight to get rid of parasitic blood vessels

Excessive body fat can raise blood pressure by offering resistance to the flow of blood. If you can "pinch up" more than one inch of fat anywhere on your body, you should begin *now* to exercise some control over your eating habits. Eliminate all foods containing white sugar or white flour. Eat only fresh, natural foods. Five or six smaller meals each day may be less fattening than the conventional three large meals a day. (See Chapter 15 for more about reducing your body weight.)

A rice diet will reduce blood pressure

A low-sodium diet of rice and fruit juice (with a vitamin and mineral supplement) is often effective in lowering blood pressure. It may not be a good idea to stay on such a low-protein diet for more than a few weeks, however, and only then with your doctor's permission.

Open up your blood vessels with garlic

Eating garlic, or swallowing garlic perles or tablets, will sometimes lower blood pressure by dilating tiny veins and arteries. Garlic certainly won't do any harm, and it is a nutritious food. If you don't want the odor of garlic on your breath, take it in tablets or perles—or mix it with plenty of parsley.

How John H. took the lid off his emotional stress

Unrelieved emotional stress is a common cause of high blood pressure. Avoid situations that subject you to humiliation or verbal abuse. Steer clear of people who take advantage of you. Expressing your anger or "speaking your piece" will temporarily relieve emotional tension. But if the overall situation isn't changed for the better, the high blood pressure will return.

Take the case of John H., for example. He was a struggling service station operator who lived with his "good-for-nothing in-laws." He had consistently high blood pressure that had totally defied all forms of treatment. Once, when he physically attacked his nagging brother-in-law, his blood pressure dropped to normal— but only for a day or two. When he finally succeeded in his business and purchased a home of his own, his blood pressure returned to normal and stayed there.

How to Cope with Low Blood Pressure and Dizzy Spells

Low blood pressure is not usually a problem unless it gets so low that fainting or dizziness occurs. When no symptoms occur, a low pressure usually favors a long life.

Many people complain of dizziness when they stand erect suddenly from a sitting or lying position. This is usually called *postural hypotension.* The sudden change in posture and the effect of gravity simply drains blood from the brain. Ordinarily, heart action and a reflex constriction of the blood vessels in the legs and the abdomen will maintain an even flow of blood to the brain, no matter what position you're in. If your circulatory system is slow in adjusting to sudden postural changes, protect yourself by getting up in stages. When you get out of bed, for example, sit on the edge of the bed for a few minutes before standing erect.

A special diet for low blood pressure

If you suffer from fatigue and weakness that you feel may be caused by low blood pressure (a systolic pressure of 90 or less), a high-protein diet might help. Plenty of chicken and fish, for example, will supply the protein and Vitamin B you need to maintain your normal blood pressure. You should avoid refined sweets and starches completely, since they satisfy your appetite without supplying all the elements you need to support your circulatory system.

How to Aid Circulation in Varicose Veins

Varicose veins occur independently of hardened arteries, although both can occur at the same time. Normally, one-way valves in the veins keep the blood flowing toward the heart. When these valves fail, the blood simply backs up in the veins under the pull of gravity, causing them to become varicose, or swollen and knotty. Varicose veins occur almost exclusively in the legs and lower abdomen where venous blood must flow uphill. (Hemorrhoids are varicose veins.)

The circulatory interference of varicose veins can cause leg fatigue, muscle cramps, swollen ankles, and leg ulcers. In severe cases, the veins may become painfully inflamed and filled with clots.

How to elevate your legs
to drain swollen veins

Unlike atherosclerosis, in which the legs must be lowered to encourage the flow of blood through clogged arteries, the legs must be *elevated* to aid circulation in varicose veins. Lying down with your feet up on a chair, or sitting with your feet higher than your hips, will drain stagnant blood out of swollen veins and reduce swollen ankles.

Becky R., who worked long hours in a busy flower shop, suffered from leg ache and swollen ankles at the end of each day. When her employer allowed her to lie down and elevate her legs several times a day, her symptoms eased considerably.

Note: Watermelon or cucumber juice, without salt added, will help remove excess fluid from swollen ankles by stimulating the kidneys. Some herbal teas are also effective diuretics. Remember that excessive use of artificial diuretics can result in a loss of potassium, which can cause symptoms of illness.

How to use a compression bandage
to prevent filling of enlarged veins

Wrapping the lower leg from the foot to the knee with a wide elastic bandage, or simply wearing elastic stockings, will keep enlarged veins compressed so that they won't collect blood and allow fluid to seep out into the tissues. Wrap your legs with a four-inch bandage, overlapping it about two inches on each turn. Make a turn or two around the ankle and under the arch before beginning a spiral up your leg. It's best to wrap both legs immediately after elevating them for a half-hour or so. When you remove the wrapping, rub your legs gently with witch hazel or rubbing alcohol.

How to pump blood with leg muscles and water pressure

Even normal veins depend largely upon the pumping action of muscular contraction for the movement of blood. In the legs where venous blood flow is hindered by the pull of gravity, regular use of leg muscles is essential. If you have a job that requires you to sit or stand for hours at a time, walk a few steps every chance you get—or at least rise up and down on your toes occasionally. Don't ever lie in bed for long periods of time without contracting the muscles in your thighs and legs.

Walking in waist-deep water (particularly salt water or mineral spring water) will relieve painful swelling in varicose veins. The buoyancy of the water aids the flow of venous blood by reducing the pull of gravity. The pressure of the water against the outside of the legs will prevent swelling of the veins. The temperature of the water, hot or cold, and the massaging effect of movement in the water will stimulate nerves as well as activate blood vessels. Combine all this with contraction of leg muscles and you have effective circulatory stimulation for arterial blood flow as well as for venous blood flow.

How to Use a "Gelatin Boot" for Speedy Healing of a Varicose Ulcer

If varicose veins result in an ulcer on your leg, you can speed healing (without going to bed) by supporting the tissues of the leg with a gelatin boot. The constant and rigid support of the boot will keep the veins compressed so that an increased flow of blood can aid nature in healing the ulcer.

Melt a couple of packages of plain gelatin in the top of a double boiler. Rub a little petrolatum or Vaseline petroleum jelly over the ulcer and cover it with a sterile gauze dressing. Then wrap the leg with a layer of gauze from the bottom of the foot to just below the knee. Make sure that the gauze isn't folded or wrinkled. Paint the gauze with a coat of warm, liquid gelatin. A two-inch paint brush should do fine. Wrap the leg with another layer of gauze and paint on another coat of gelatin. Repeat this procedure three or four times, finishing with a heavy coat of gelatin. Leave the boot on for about six days. Continue walking in your normal activities so that contraction of the leg muscles will aid the circulation of blood.

When the gelatin boot is removed, wash the leg with soap and water and carefully apply rubbing alcohol. If the ulcer hasn't healed, you can wait a day or two and apply another boot. Or you may simply rest in bed and cleanse the ulcer daily with soap and water. Towels wrung out in warm, salty water and applied over the ulcer will stimulate healing. If swelling is present, elevate the foot of the bed three or four inches. When the ulcer has healed, you should continue to wear elastic bandages or stockings to aid venous circulation and to prevent a recurrence of the ulcer.

How to use a simple rubber-and-bandage wrapping for small ulcers

An effect similar to that of a gelatin boot can be obtained with a special wrapping. Cover the ulcer with sterile petrolatum (Vaseline petroleum jelly, etc.) and gauze, and then cover the gauze with sponge rubber that's about three-quarters of an inch thick and large enough to extend one inch beyond the ulcer margin. Over this, snugly wrap an elastic adhesive bandage that extends about two inches above and below the ulcer. Change the dressing once or twice a week for one to three weeks.

A contrast bath will benefit varicose ulcers

Immersing the affected leg knee-deep in hot water for one minute and in ice water for one minute, for a total time of about

20 minutes, will speed the healing of a varicose ulcer. Remember, however, that you cannot use such extreme temperatures if you are also suffering from hardened arteries.

How to Relieve the Agony of Phlebitis

If your leg veins become inflamed and obstructed, causing swelling, pain, and muscle tenderness, you should go to bed and keep your legs slightly elevated for at least six days. A cradle over your legs will prevent irritation by bed covers. Mildly warm or cool compresses, whichever feels best, may be used to relieve pain and stimulate circulation.

If the symptoms subside after six days, wrap your legs lightly with an elastic bandage and begin moving around slowly and progressively. Contraction of the leg muscles while the legs are wrapped will aid circulation. Continue to wear the bandage as long as necessary to prevent a recurrence of swelling.

Several hundred units of Vitamin E daily, taken orally, will help dissolve clots in clogged veins.

Summary

1. Lecithin, vegetable oil, Vitamin E, the B vitamins, and a diet low in animal fat will relieve symptoms caused by hard fat and cholesterol that have accumulated in your arteries.
2. Contraction of leg muscles while the legs are in a lowered position aids circulation in hardened arteries below the knee.
3. An ounce or two of whiskey or brandy will relieve the leg pain caused by spasm of blood vessels during the night.
4. A carbon dioxide bath in your own home will ease the workload on your heart by dilating blood vessels and normalizing your blood pressure.
5. You shouldn't apply heat to legs that have been crippled by hardened arteries, but you *can* improve circulation in such legs by applying heat to the abdomen.
6. A drink made by soaking hawthorn berries in boiling water is believed to be effective in relieving heart pain by dilating the coronary arteries.
7. If you have high blood pressure, you should go easy on salt,

coffee, cigarettes, and increase your intake of garlic, fresh fruit, and seafood.

8. You can drain swollen varicose veins by elevating your legs, which should be followed by wrapping with a wide elastic bandage or support with elastic hose.

9. A gelatin boot applied at home is often very effective in speeding recovery from ulcers caused by varicose veins.

10. Phlebitis should be treated initially with bed rest, elevation of the legs, and warm or cool compresses, followed by use of a compression bandage to prevent a recurrence of swelling.

2

Naturomatic Healing Methods for Coughs, Colds, Sore Throat, and Other Respiratory Ailments

There's an old saying to the effect that "you don't appreciate it until you've lost it." For most of us, breathing is such a natural, automatic process that we give little thought to the act of breathing. Yet there are many thousands of people who must struggle for every breath they take. Few of us can imagine what it's like not to be able to get enough oxygen or to take a deep, satisfying breath. With the spread of air pollution, however, and the increasing threat of allergic reactions to foreign chemicals in the foods we eat, not to mention the lowered resistance that results from poor health, the chances are great that all of us will eventually suffer from some type of respiratory trouble.

Just about everyone suffers from colds, coughs, sore throat, and other infections of the respiratory tract. The use of natural remedies in the care of these ailments will give you a solid foundation for coping with the more uncommon ailments. There's plenty that you can do to relieve all types of respiratory ailments—and you can use remedies that can be applied right in your own home. This chapter tells you how.

How to Relieve the Symptoms of Emphysema

Emphysema is the fastest-growing disease in the United States. It is already becoming a leading cause of death and disability.

When this dreaded disease strikes, the air sacs of the lungs become hard and enlarged, so that they cannot empty the air they contain when you exhale. This means that you cannot breathe out enough stale air to make room for fresh air. As a result, the slightest amount of physical exertion causes an agonizing shortness of breath that literally cripples your body. Mucus may accumulate in your bronchial tubes causing a chronic cough. When emphysema becomes advanced, you must struggle constantly for breath. Carbon dioxide waste accumulates in your blood and poisons your tissues. An oxygen deficiency results in an increased production of red blood cells, causing your blood to become thick and syrupy. All of this places considerable strain on your heart. Resistance is also lowered, so that frequent chest colds occur.

If you're over forty years of age and you suffer from breathlessness and a chronic cough, there's a good chance that you might be suffering from emphysema, even if it cannot be detected by X-ray examination. A person who is not physically active may lose 50 percent of his lung tissue before he begins to experience symptoms of emphysema.

The match test for emphysema

Hold a lighted match out at arm's length. If you have emphysema, you'll find it difficult or impossible to blow out the flame.

How to moisturize the air you breathe

Ordinarily, the air you exhale pushes mucus out of your lungs so that it can be coughed up and "spit out." When your lungs have been damaged by emphysema, however, inability to exhale forcefully allows mucus to accumulate in your bronchial tubes. The air you breathe then absorbs moisture from the mucus, leaving it dry and sticky. This clogs bronchial tubes and causes a chronic, dry cough that may aggravate emphysema by rupturing hardened air sacs. For this reason, you should humidify or moisturize the air you breathe in order to soften the mucus in your lungs so that it can be expelled.

Moisture can be added to the air with commercial vaporizers or by boiling a pot of water on the stove. Many people add humidifiers to central furnaces and air conditioners. During the winter, some simply keep a pan of water on top of a room heater. Inhaling steam in a hot shower is an effective way to loosen mucus. It might be a good idea to purchase a pocket nebulizer that mixes water and air into an aerosol that can be inhaled at will.

How to empty your bronchial tubes with postural drainage

After breathing steam or water vapor, you should pound your chest with your fingertips to break loose stubborn mucus. Lying first on one side and then on the other will move mucus from the smaller tubes into the larger tubes. Then lie across a bed with the upper half of your body hanging over the side of the bed so that both of your forearms are resting on the floor. This will place your lungs in an upside-down position so that you can cough up all the loose mucus. Place a basin close by your head so that you won't have to get up to expectorate. (See Figure 1.)

Postural drainage is particularly effective in bronchiectasis, in which large amounts of mucus and pus are coughed up from infected bronchial tubes.

How to combine breathing and walking to relieve breathlessness

After your lungs have been cleaned with postural drainage and you're able to breathe better, it might be a good idea to take a walk and practice deep breathing exercises. When the weather is very cold, however, you may have to exercise in a warm, humidified room rather than walk outdoors. Extremely cold air is usually very dry and will absorb an excessive amount of moisture from your lungs.

Regular walking and breathing exercises will condition your muscles and your heart so that you can do more with less oxygen. This means that even if emphysema has destroyed a large portion of your lung tissue, you can live a normal life if you are in good physical condition.

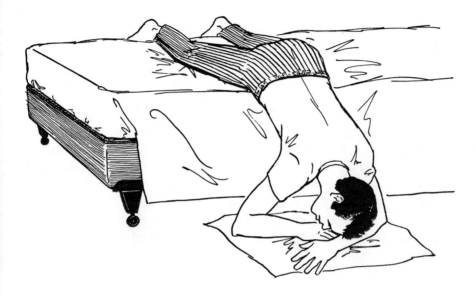

Drawing by Bibiana Neal

Figure 1. Position for draining mucus and phlegm from the body.

Walter C., for example, a 60-year-old emphysemic who couldn't walk 20 feet without losing his breath, was able to go back to his surveying business after several months of cleaning out his lungs and taking regular walks. On cold, dry days, rather than skip his exercise, he rode a stationary bicycle in his humidified bedroom.

Occasionally lie down on the floor and breathe deeply into your abdomen (making a pot belly) in order to train your diaphragm for more efficient breathing.

How to empty your lungs
with positive pressure breathing

Exhaling forcefully through pursed lips or through a small drinking straw will force expansion of collapsed bronchioles (tiny air passages) so that you can empty your lungs more completely without rupturing damaged air sacs.

A better diet for faster healing of lungs

Good nutrition is just as important in the treatment of emphysema as it is in the treatment of any other disease. You *must* have a diet of fresh, natural foods, and you should increase your intake of Vitamins A and C in order to build healthy lung tissue that will resist infection. Remember that any kind of respiratory infection can be serious for persons suffering from emphysema. A Vitamin E supplement will increase your endurance and reduce your body's need for oxygen. (Don't smoke cigarettes—and stay out of smoke-filled rooms. You can't possibly get enough oxygen if you fill your lungs with smoke and load your red blood cells with carbon monoxide.)

Drink plenty of liquids—preferably fruit and vegetable juices and water—to increase the amount of moisture eliminated through your lungs. Even if you humidify the air in your home, it can hold only a certain amount of moisture at a certain temperature. If the temperature of the air is less than your body temperature, as it should be, the air will absorb moisture while it's in your lungs.

Hints for Victims of Asthma, Hay Fever, and Other Allergies

Remove irritating elements from the air you breathe

Asthma, or spasm of tiny air passages, can be caused by infection, but it's most commonly caused by an allergy. So the first thing you should do in the treatment of asthma and other respiratory allergies is to remove fumes, dust, pollen, or any other irritating element, including cigarette smoke, from the air you breathe. All types of air-borne matter—from insect spray to dog dandruff—can trigger an allergic reaction in the bronchial tubes.

Try to keep the air in your home as free from floating particles as possible. Get rid of old rugs, ancient upholstered furniture, venetian blinds, lined drapes, vases, "whatnots," and other "dust catchers." Have your home vacuumed frequently. Put airtight covers on pillows, cushions, and mattresses. Filter the air of your bedroom with air conditioning in the summer. If you use gas units to heat your rooms in the winter, make sure that the heaters are vented to the outside. Vents should also be placed over cooking stoves. You'll be able to think of many things that you can do to keep dust and fumes from polluting the air in your home. If you suffer from *seasonal* allergies, you'll know that you're probably sensitive to pollen that must be filtered out of the air you breathe.

Check your diet for food allergies

Every time you have an attack of asthma or hay fever, try to determine whether you have eaten, breathed, or come into contact with anything that might have resulted in an allergic reaction. If you have difficulty breathing after mixing whole wheat flour or after cleaning out the attic, you won't need a doctor to tell you that you're suffering from an allergy. Some cosmetics contain orris root, rice powder, or corn starch, which can trigger an allergic reaction in some people.

If you suspect that you might be allergic to something you're eating, try eliminating the suspected foods from your diet—one at a time—until you note an improvement in your condition. Eggs, wheat, milk, and chocolate commonly result in allergic reactions.

How to correct
nutritional deficiencies

No one knows for sure why some people are allergic to some things and other people are not. There is some evidence, however, to indicate that poor health or a nutritional deficiency is often a factor. So if you have asthma or hay fever, or any other type of allergy, switch to a good, balanced diet of fresh, natural foods. Such a diet will improve digestion and elimination as well as supply the nutrients your body needs to heal itself.

Remember that *all* the essential vitamins and minerals work together in overcoming infections and allergies. Eat some of all the basic foods each day. According to the Department of Agriculture, there are four main classes of food: meat, vegetables and fruits, milk and milk products, and whole grain bread and cereals. If you find that you are allergic to milk and milk products, be sure to take a good calcium supplement (along with Vitamin D). Persons who are allergic to wheat should take Vitamin E. A little extra Vitamin C will do wonders in helping your body overcome tissue reactions in allergies.

How to control allergies by controlling your blood sugar

It's now well known that hypoglycemia or low blood sugar is a common cause of all types of allergies, including asthma. This is why asthma can sometimes be temporarily relieved by eating sweets or by injecting drugs such as adrenalin that raise blood sugar. Few people know, however, that eating refined sugar can actually *lower* blood sugar by triggering an insulin reaction four to six hours after eating.

The parents of an overweight 10-year-old boy reported that the lad frequently had attacks of asthma in the middle of the night. A study of his eating habits revealed that he was constantly eating candy and drinking soda pop, and that his meals were rich in refined carbohydrates. When he switched to natural foods and started snacking on fruits and nuts, *his asthma disappeared.* His "food allergies" also disappeared, and his body weight dropped to a normal level. Apparently, the boy's blood sugar had been falling during the night because of pancreatic reaction to an excessive sugar intake during the day.

How to relieve asthma by controlling your emotions

Prolonged emotional stress can cause asthma and other allergies by exhausting the adrenal glands. You'll learn in the next chapter how to control stress and ease tensions.

Even when asthma isn't caused by stress, it can be severely

aggravated by emotional excitement, turning a mild attack into a medical emergency. So try not to panic during an asthmatic attack. Get into a position that seems most comfortable and relax. Remember that uncomplicated asthma is rarely fatal. You should, of course, seek medical aid when the disease is severe or if you have heart trouble.

You can exhale easier with
a bottle of water

During the attack of asthma, try exhaling forcefully through a drinking straw that has been inserted into a large bottle of water. The resistance of the water will force expansion of spastic bronchial tubes by creating positive pressure in your lungs. In other words, an increase in pressure inside your bronchial tubes will hold tiny air passages open while your breathing muscles force stale air out of your lungs. You may then fill your lungs with fresh air.

How to Take Effective Action Against the Common Cold

You've heard it said many times that there is no cure for a cold. This is true when it comes to drugs and patent medicines. There is, however, a great deal that you can do to relieve symptoms and speed recovery from a cold. In fact, if you don't take steps to aid your body in overcoming a cold infection, the lowered resistance that results could lead to pneumonia, bronchitis, and other serious infections that can contribute to the development of emphysema, asthma, allergies, and other chronic ailments.

Increase your intake of Vitamin C

When you first begin to feel the dry scratchy throat that usually precedes a cold, start taking Vitamin C tablets along with increased quantities of fruit juice. Take 300 to 500 milligrams every hour for several hours. If no side effects occur (such as diarrhea) and the cold does not let up, you can increase the dosage the second day. It's better to take frequent small doses than to take only a few large doses. Too large a dose at one time results in loss of the vitamin through the kidneys. Also, infrequent doses do not keep the tissues saturated for constant defense against cold germs. *You should take Vitamin C at least every four hours to replenish that lost in fighting infection.* It may not be a good idea, however, for a healthy person to take extra large doses of the vitamin over a long period of time, since elimination of the vitamin through the kidneys may lead to bladder irritation.

The Food and Nutrition Board of the National Research Council recommends 60 milligrams of Vitamin C per day for healthy men. There are some researchers, however, who say that we need as much as 2,000 milligrams a day during the cold season when fresh fruits and vegetables are not plentiful.

Note: Nicotine from cigarettes destroys Vitamin C in the blood. If you smoke, you need more Vitamin C than a nonsmoker.

Bathe your throat with acid vapor

The secretions of the nose are normally slightly acid, but when a cold begins they become alkaline and the throat becomes dry. Bathing the throat and nasal passages with an acid vapor will moisten the throat and kill the germs that haven't already embedded themselves in the mucus membranes. Put just enough vinegar in a pot of boiling water to give off a comfortably acid vapor. Inhale the vapor at the first sign of a cold.

Kill cold germs
with garlic and onion

Garlic is a potent germicide that you can use to kill cold germs if you—and the people around you—can stand the odor. Put garlic on your food during the cold season. When a cold first begins, eat a little chopped garlic and parsley. In addition to being rich in Vitamin C and iron, the parsley will help neutralize the strong odor of the garlic.

The Swiss immerse a slice of raw onion in a glass of hot water and then sip the water for cold protection.

Control the temperature and humidity
of your home

Going out into the cold from a hot room may be a major factor in delaying recovery from winter colds. Keep the temperature in your home below 75 degrees. If there is adequate moisture in the air of your home, a temperature of 72 degrees Fahrenheit will be warm enough for you. You should be able to sit around the house in light clothing without any discomfort.

Humidify the air of your home so that the relative humidity is at least 45 percent. A high degree of moisture keeps down cold germs and keeps your mucous membranes moist enough to resist further infection. Placing a pot of water on top of a heater or stove is a simple way to moisturize the air. Potted plants in your home will give off oxygen and water vapor.

You can measure the amount of moisture in the air with a psychrometer, a device that contains a wet bulb and a dry bulb thermometer. There are many moderately priced humidity indicators on the market.

General measures to relieve
a clogged or dry nose
and other symptoms

Get a little rest, increase your intake of fluids, and avoid chills. Inhale steam vapor to loosen the mucus in your nose and then blow both nostrils at the same time. Leave your mouth open and do not blow too forcefully. "Honking" your nose, or blowing one nostril at a time, may force cold germs into your inner ear or into your sinuses.

If the membrane in your nose becomes dry and cracked, rub a little vegetable oil, Vaseline petroleum jelly, or glycerin up in your nose with your finger. It's especially important to oil the membranes of the nose when heated air lacks adequate moisture. Don't use oil in place of nose drops, however. If a drop of oil gets into your lungs, a serious form of pneumonia could result.

Don't be tempted by commercial "cold remedies." Such medicines will only suppress symptoms and delay recovery. The only way to get rid of a cold safely and quickly is to help your body cure itself.

How to Soothe a Sore Throat and Cope with Tonsillitis

When simple sore throat strikes, a hot gargle will wash away germs and stimulate circulation for soothing relief and a speedy recovery. Mix half a teaspoon of table salt to a glass of hot water (about 110 degrees Fahrenheit). Gargle several times a day.

If gargling makes you gag, you can irrigate your throat by dropping your chin down on your chest and using a syringe or rubber bulb to squirt warm, salty water against the back of your throat. Leave your mouth open so that the water can run out freely into a basin—and keep your throat closed so that you won't swallow any of the salt water.

Note: Gargling with water containing a little bicarbonate of soda will help clear mucus out of the throat.

How to relieve a sore throat with
hot drinks and seaweed lemonade

Hot drinks will soothe a sore throat that cannot be reached by gargling or irrigating. *Irish moss lemonade* makes a thick, syrupy drink that coats the throat for long-lasting relief. Wash a quarter of a cup of Irish moss and let it soak for 15 minutes. Drain the water, add two cups of cold water, and cook in the top of a double boiler until the concoction becomes syrupy. Strain the liquid and then add four tablespoons of lemon juice and enough honey to suit your taste.

Irish moss, also called *carrageen,* is a dried seaweed that can be purchased in health food stores.

How to use fomentations
for a sore throat

Apply a large fomentation to the throat and upper chest while the feet are soaking in a pan of hot water. Material that is about 50 percent cotton and 50 percent wool will hold moisture and heat best. A piece of part-woolen gown or blanket, or even an old undershirt, will suffice. Just wring the material out in hot water, cover it with a piece of dry flannel to conserve heat and to prevent a burn, and then place over the throat and chest. Renew the fomentation every few minutes for at least three applications. At the end of the treatment, rub the throat with a cold wash cloth. Dry the feet and put on a pair of warm woolen socks.

Two or three times a day, alternate the application of hot cloths and cold cloths, three changes each, for circulatory stimulation.

An overnight heating compress
for sore throat

Cut three strips of cotton cloth about three inches wide and long enough to wrap around your throat twice. Cut two strips of flannel the same length and at least four inches wide. Wring the cotton cloths out in cold water (60 degrees F.) and wrap them around your neck. Then wrap the flannel around your neck and pin it in place. Make sure that the moist cloth is completely covered by the flannel.

The compress will feel cold at first, but the moist cloth will be quickly warmed by your body. Leave the compress on overnight; then remove it and rub your neck with cold water.

How to use hot packs and cold packs
to relieve tonsillitis

A sore throat with painful swelling on one or both sides of the throat may mean tonsillitis. Apply *hot* moist cloths (wrapped in flannel) to both sides of the throat for five minutes, followed by an *ice bag* for five minutes, with three changes of each, two or three times a day. Follow each treatment with a cold neck rub.

A heating compress, such as that recommended for overnight use in the treatment of a sore throat, may be used between treatments.

A 20-year-old nurse's aid was suddenly stricken with acute tonsillitis that was accompanied by a temperature of 103.5 degrees. The first treatment with hot cloths and ice bags, as described above, almost completely relieved the pain. After applying the treatment twice a day for three days, her temperature was back to normal and the soreness was nearly gone.

How to Get Quick Relief for Inflammation of the
Nose, Throat, Sinuses, and Chest

How to use medicated steam
for aggravating coughs

For uncomplicated coughs, croup, bronchitis, laryngitis, and sinusitis, boil a pot of water and inhale the steam for 20 to 30 minutes. A teaspoonful of menthol, oil of eucalyptus, camphor, or oil of pine added to the water will provide more soothing relief. You can drape a large towel over your head to form a tent or canopy that will catch the steam so that you won't have to lean directly over the boiling water. If you prefer, you can inhale the steam through a large paper cone. If you want to lie down while inhaling steam, lie next to a vaporizer, place a large umbrella on the floor above your head, and then have someone cover the whole works with a sheet.

Keeping a pan of water on top of your heater during the winter is often very effective in relieving a cough caused by chronic bronchitis or a tracheal (windpipe) irritation. A housewife who suffered from a cough that lasted for six weeks every winter obtained complete relief for the first time in ten years after putting a pan of water on top of a space heater. The increased amount of moisture in the air simply prevented drying and irritation of the membranes of her nose and throat.

How to use cold packs and hot foot baths
to relieve acute sinusitis

When the hollow, bony cavities in the bones of your face become acutely inflamed, infected, or clogged, the pain that results may not be relieved with simple steam inhalations. In fact, the application of heat may sometimes increase the pain. Whenever this happens, you should place a cold pack over the painful sinuses while your feet are immersed in a pan of hot water. This will relieve pressure in the sinuses by decreasing the flow of blood in the swollen membranes that line the sinus cavities. The hot foot bath will draw blood to the feet, while the cold pack over the face will drive blood out of the sinuses by contracting blood vessels.

You can make an effective cold pack by putting crushed ice in a sealed plastic bag and then wrapping the bag in a slightly moist towel.

How to unclog your nose
and sinuses with irrigation

Inhaling steam will usually open your nose and your sinuses. When the nose is clogged with thick mucus and crust, however, it might help to irrigate your nose.

Attach a couple inches of rubber tubing to a funnel and then attach a large medicine dropper to the end of the tubing. Mix half a teaspoon of salt into about three ounces of warm water. Pinch the tubing shut and pour the water into the funnel. Lie down on one side, place the dropper in the uppermost nostril, and let the water run from one nostril to the other while you breathe through your mouth. If the water doesn't seem to get through the passages that connect both sides of the nose, lie on the opposite side and try the opposite nostril. If you prefer, you may simply put the water up in your nose with an eye dropper. After the irrigation, wait about three minutes before blowing your nose.

A gentle suction up in the nose with a syringe will sometimes help remove sticky plugs in the sinus openings.

How onion can clean your nose

Some folk healers maintain that smelling a freshly cut onion will open clogged nasal passages. Onion, like garlic, contains a substance that tends to kill bacteria. Simply peeling an onion will start a flow of tears that will often open a clogged nose.

How to use a penetrating mustard
plaster for chest soreness

A mustard plaster laid over the chest will relieve irritation and congestion deep within the chest by combining moist heat with counter-irritation. You can purchase a ready-made mustard plaster in a drug store, or you can make your own.

To make a mustard plaster for adults, mix one part table mustard (or powdered mustard) with four to six parts of flour (12 parts flour for children) and mix in *slightly warm* water to make a smooth paste. Then spread the mixture about a quarter of an inch thick over a piece of muslin that's large enough to cover the chest. Cover the plaster with another piece of muslin and fold the edges over to prevent leakage. When the plaster is placed on the chest, cover it with wax paper or oil cloth.

Remove the plaster from the chest when the skin begins to redden—usually after five to 20 minutes. Wash the skin with warm soap and water, dry it with a towel, and then oil the skin slightly before covering with warm flannel.

Note: If mustard is exposed to a temperature greater than 140 degrees Fahrenheit, it will not release the oil that is responsible for the healing effect.

How to Relieve Lung Congestion Caused by Respiratory Infection

Chest congestion caused by influenza, bronchitis, pneumonia, and colds can be relieved by fomentations or moist heat applications applied to the chest while the feet are immersed in hot water.

Place a wash tub or a deep pan on the bed and fill it about half full of hot water. Then lie down on the bed, bend your knees, and place your feet in the water. A member of the family can keep the water hot by occasionally adding a little hot faucet water. Make sure that the water is not hotter than 115 degrees. Oil of wintergreen or a tablespoonful of mustard may be added to the water to intensify the heating action.

Fomentations can be made by wringing out a folded part-woolen cloth in hot water and then wrapping it in a piece of dry flannel before applying it to the chest. The whole body—moist packs and all—should be covered with blankets to induce sweating. Sipping hot lemonade will hasten sweating. When the body temperature is excessive, a moist, cold towel applied to the head during the treatment will relieve discomfort.

Change the chest fomentation every five or ten minutes for at least three applications. Be sure to dry the skin between applications so that moisture accumulating on the skin won't result in a burn.

At the conclusion of the treatment, the body should be rubbed with a moist, cold wash cloth or a towel-mitten to restore normal vascular tone. Uncover only one body part at a time for the cold rub, however, and then dry and cover the part before going on to the next part. Don't discontinue the foot bath or the chest fomentation until the cold rub is nearly completed. It's important to avoid chilling.

How to Ease the Stabbing Pain of Pleurisy

Pleurisy is a chest pain that makes breathing painful and a deep breath impossible. The symptoms result from a rubbing between inflamed membranes that line the space between the chest walls and the lungs.

A hot foot bath followed by three to five moist heat applications over the painful area will usually relieve the pain. Wring out a part-woolen cloth in 110-degree water, lay it over a piece of dry flannel over the chest, and then cover it with another piece of dry flannel. Change the application every five minutes until the pain eases. Do this twice a day for a couple of days. After each treatment, dry the skin and wrap the chest in warm flannel. When the feet are removed from the hot foot bath, rub them with a cool cloth or pour a dipper of cool water over them.

Wrapping the chest *tightly* with the wide strips of flannel will reduce pain by restricting rib movement. You can buy special rib belts (in any drug store) that can be used to strap down the ribs.

Cold applications should not be applied over the chest in the treatment of pleurisy. But once the acute pain is gone, it might help to alternate a hot, moist cloth with a cool, moist cloth for circulatory stimulation.

How Billy J. handled his
pleurisy attack

Billy J., a telephone linesman, developed a severe breathing pain in the right side of his chest after being chilled by a cold wind.

When examination revealed the presence of pleurisy, a hot foot bath was given, followed by four fomentations (moist-heat applications) over the entire right side of his chest. After this, the skin was dried and covered with warmed flannel. Twice during the night, an electric heating pad was applied over the painful area for about half an hour. Treatment was applied twice a day for three days. By the end of the third day, Billy J. could breathe much better and the pain was nearly gone.

How to Reduce a Fever

Cold drinks, cold compresses applied to the head and neck, a cold-water enema, sponging with cool water or alcohol, or rubbing ice over the spine will reduce excessive body temperature. One ounce of menthol liniment mixed with three or four ounces of water also has a cooling effect when rubbed on the skin.

Remember, however, that *fever is part of nature's defense against infection.* So don't be concerned about getting rid of low fevers. The only thing you want to do is to help dissipate excessive heat in *high* fevers. Use cold applications only when body temperature is uncomfortably high (causing headache, insomnia, and other symptoms) and the skin is hot and dry. You shouldn't allow your temperature to go above 105 degrees Fahrenheit. Some doctors believe that an oral temperature above 104 degrees is harmful. (Oral temperature is one degree lower than rectal temperature.) Victims of heat stroke are very often immersed in cold water to keep their rectal temperature from going above 105 degrees.

When fever is accompanied by chills or a cold, clammy skin, it would be better to sponge the skin with warm water to induce sweating.

In everyday fevers and infections, plenty of fresh, cool fruit or vegetable juice will provide cooling nourishment that will combat infection and maintain the alkali reserve of the blood.

How to Care for Diaphragmatic Hernia

In an esophageal hiatus diaphragmatic hernia, a portion of the stomach protrudes up into the chest through an opening in the diaphragm. It usually causes chest and upper abdominal pain and belching (and sometimes hiccups) that occur after eating. The remedy is to eat small meals and to avoid lying down immediately after eating. If you should lose control of your taste buds and overindulge on a special occasion, you may have to sleep sitting up to avoid heartburn and respiratory distress. Avoid spicy and coarse foods that might cause irritation if they are trapped in the stomach above the diaphragm.

Sylvia G. had been complaining of chest pains for several years. Doctors had assured her that her heart was normal. "It sometimes feels as if I have a giant air bubble in the center of my chest," she said with obvious anxiety. "And no matter how hard I try, I just cannot belch it up. It gets worse when I lie down, especially after I eat."

Sylvia had a diaphragmatic hernia. When she overate, food trapped in the portion of the stomach above her diaphragm triggered a spasm that could not be relieved by belching. She got complete relief by eating smaller meals consisting of natural, unseasoned foods, by reducing her body weight, and by elevating the head of her bed with eight-inch blocks.

Note: Diaphragmatic hernias are often complicated by stomach ulcers. If you have heartburn or a burning stomach pain, see Chapter 9 for ulcer remedies.

How to Control Nervous Breathing and Hiccups

If you suffer from dizziness, faintness, numbness, tingling, headache, and other symptoms that seem to be associated with nervousness and inability to get enough oxygen, you might be hyperventilating. This means that excessive deep breathing is siphoning too much carbon dioxide out of your blood, thus upsetting the chemical control of the breathing centers in your brain. The next time you start gasping for breath or breathing rapidly because of nervousness, you may be able to control your respiration by fitting a medium size paper bag over your mouth and nose and breathing the air in the bag over and over for a few minutes.

How to Eliminate the Causes of Bad Breath

According to mouthwash ads on television, all that's needed for success in love and business is a sweet-smelling breath! True or not, the ads do reflect widespread concern about a common problem. Don't be misled, however, into thinking that the answer to bad breath lies solely in mouthwashes and candy tablets. Such measures simply mask the odor, which returns again in a very short while. The only way to get rid of bad breath permanently is to eliminate the source of the odor.

Clean out your mouth

Most bad breath originates in the mouth. Food particles trapped between the teeth and under the edge of the gums begin to decompose less than half an hour after eating, giving off a bad odor. The remedy for this is to brush your teeth after each meal and use dental floss each night before retiring. If you eat anything between meals, rinse your mouth and teeth with water. Force the water between your teeth by squishing it back and forth.

If bad breath persists in spite of thorough cleaning of your teeth, have a dentist check your gums. You may have hidden pockets around the roots of your teeth where food particles rot undisturbed.

Brush your tongue

Take a look at your tongue. If it appears to be coated, stick it out and brush it with your tooth brush. The tongue is covered with tiny, fleshy buds and grooves that can trap food particles quite easily. Without proper cleansing, your tongue can get quite coated.

Balance the bacterial content
of your intestinal tract

In some cases, bad breath can be caused by gasses that have been absorbed from the intestinal tract and eliminated through the lungs. If your stool has a foul odor, intestinal putrefaction may be contributing to bad breath. Yogurt, or milk containing acidophilus culture, will aid digestion and destroy the putrefactive bacteria in your colon. You can purchase acidophilus culture in drug stores and health food stores.

Summary

1. If you are suffering from emphysema, you must moisturize the air you breathe, drain mucus out of your bronchial tubes, and build resistance against respiratory infection.
2. Asthma is most often an allergy caused by house dust, fumes, and other impurities in the air.
3. Exhaling forcefully through a small drinking straw into a large bottle of water may relieve an asthmatic attack by forcing expansion of spastic bronchial tubes.
4. Low blood sugar, caused by eating sugar and other refined carbohydrates, is commonly an indirect cause of all types of allergies.
5. You may be able to abort or shorten the course of a cold by taking heavy doses of Vitamin C, by eating garlic and onion, or by inhaling steam from water that has been mixed with vinegar.
6. Bad breath almost always originates in the mouth, and can usually be eliminated by cleaning the tongue as well as the teeth.
7. A hot salt-water gargle or irrigation, or a hot drink, will soothe a sore throat. Tonsillitis, however, may be best relieved by alternating hot and cold applications to the outside of the throat.
8. Inhaling steam containing menthol, camphor, or oil of eucalyptus will provide soothing relief for coughs, bronchitis, croup, sinusitis, and laryngitis.
9. Moist heat applied to the chest while the feet are immersed in hot water will relieve pain and congestion in respiratory infections.
10. A painful sinus infection can sometimes be relieved by applying a cold pack to the face while the feet are immersed in hot water.

3

How to Cope with Disease More Successfully by Relieving Everyday Stress and Tension with Naturomatic Healing

More than a hundred years ago, Thoreau wrote that "The mass of men lead lives of quiet desperation." Today, this observation is more appropriate than ever. With a faster pace of living, a greater need for money, and longer, noisier days, the stress of life places much greater strain on the mind and emotions of man. In fact, *stress is now believed to be one of the major causes of disease.*

According to Dr. Hans Selye,* a foremost authority on the effects of stress, failure to adapt to stress, or a breakdown in the body's defense against stress, can be a factor in the development of diseases such as high blood pressure, diseases of the heart and blood vessels, diseases of the kidney, eclampsia, rheumatic and rheumatoid arthritis, inflammatory diseases of the skin and eyes, infections, allergic and hypersensitivity diseases, nervous and mental diseases, stomach ulcers, sexual derangements, digestive diseases, metabolic diseases (such as diabetes, gout, and hyperthyroidism), cancer, diseases of resistance in general, and many other types of diseases.

---

*The Stress of Life, McGraw-Hill Book Company, New York, 1956.

In my office, I frequently see patients suffering from backache, headache, myositis, fibromyositis, and other mechanical disorders that I feel are caused by prolonged muscular tension. Many doctors now believe that *almost any type of disorder can be caused by stress*—and I agree. This means that when you use natural methods to relieve the agonies of stress, you'll be able to relieve or cure a great variety of ailments that won't respond to any other form of therapy.

The programs in this chapter offer natural aids for controlling stress and tension without the use of dangerous or habit-forming drugs.

The Everyday Symptoms of Stress

When stress begins to affect the body, there may be many warning symptoms. "Heartburn," an increase in blood pressure, chest pain, headache, a skin rash, backache, a stiff neck, an aching throat, difficulty in swallowing, gas pains, upset stomach, excessive perspiration, insomnia, nervous shaking, sexual impotency, and other symptoms that seem to occur without cause may be the forerunners of disease caused by stress. When you begin to experience such symptoms, it's time to do something about the stress that's on its way to causing a "string" of diseases.

How a school teacher relieved her aches and pains by relieving her stress

Ann E. was a school teacher who complained of a variety of aches and pains. Her head hurt, her back ached, and she had abdominal pains that had defied the attempts of dozens of doctors to diagnose them. No matter what type of treatment she tried, her condition remained unchanged. It soon became apparent to me that her trouble was psychosomatic, or mentally caused. She was sick all right, but only because she couldn't cope with the discipline problems of teaching small children. She lost so much time at work that she was eventually fired from her teaching position. When she went to work in a real estate office, her pains disappeared. Had her stress continued unrelieved, she would have eventually developed serious organic disease.

The case of Gordon S.

Gordon S., one of my patients, developed a stomach ulcer after 20 years in what he thought was a degrading position that offered no hope for advancement. He finally had to submit to surgery for relief of his pain. When the ulcer began to recur, he came to me for instruction in the same tension-relieving techniques that I will describe in this chapter. The last time I saw Gordon S., he still had the same job, but his stomach ulcer was no longer bothering him.

**How one patient relieved six
different ailments with only two
natural remedies**

The case of Susan R. is a good example of how stress-caused ailments can be relieved with tension-relief programs carried out at home. She came into my office complaining of backache, but in taking her case history I learned that she also suffered from high blood pressure, an undiagnosed skin disorder, chronic diarrhea, arthritis, and headaches that were occasionally so severe that she had to be hospitalized. Yet, no doctor had been able to help her, much less cure her. She was not suffering from any obvious organic disease. She did, however, have an elevated serum cholesterol and a high uric acid, which were probably contributing to her high blood pressure and arthritic pains. She also had many personal problems that could not be resolved or forgotten.

Although I could do nothing to ease Susan's personal problems and erase her bad memories, I did recommend that she take certain measures to correct nutritional deficiencies and to combat her tension. The results were spectacular. A reduction in her serum cholesterol and uric acid lowered her blood pressure and relieved her joint pains. A Vitamin C supplement eliminated her skin disorder. Relaxation of the muscles in her neck cured her headache. "Even my stomach has settled down," she said. "And I no longer have to camp near a bathroom door."

Stress was the cause of *all* Susan's ailments. Even her Vitamin C deficiency was a result of stress. If you, too, must contend with excessive stress, you must at least do something to relieve the effects of stress. Otherwise, a vicious cycle of stress and poor health will make you progressively more ill.

How to "Breathe and Flop" to Relieve Tension

Whenever you begin to feel tension building, lie down on the floor and take several deep breaths—until you feel slightly dizzy from hyperventilation. Then lift your arms and your knees a few inches and let them flop to the floor in a totally relaxed manner. (When you lift your knees, do so without lifting your heels from the floor.) The jarring effect on your arms and the back of your knees when they strike the floor will relax muscles and produce a tingling warmth in your limbs. Concentrate on relaxing the muscles of your face and neck while you repeatedly lift and drop your arms and your knees.

If you can learn to relax your muscles so that your body is as limp as a dish rag, you can break a stress and tension cycle almost at will. Hyperventilating before attempting to relax your muscles will promote relaxation by intoxicating your brain with an imbalance of carbon dioxide and oxygen. After a couple of minutes of muscle flopping, lie relaxed on the floor for several minutes.

Relieving stress cures ulcers and colitis

An air force supply officer who suffered from peptic ulcers and colitis that resulted from overwork and constant harassment (at home as well as at work) tried the breathe-and-flop technique in his office twice a day for several weeks and reported that his digestive troubles had nearly disappeared. "I can now eat just about anything I want without any trouble," he happily reported. "Of course, I eat only natural foods as you suggested."

In my book *A Chiropractor's Treasury of Health Secrets* (Parker Publishing Company), I devoted an entire chapter to a part-by-part relaxing technique that begins with the muscles of the face and ends with the muscles of the feet. You might want to try it.

The Elephant Swing Relieves Tension and Tight Muscles

If you have ever been to a zoo, you've probably noticed that the elephants sway from side to side when they are forced to stand in a small cage. This rhythmical swaying relaxes their ponderous muscles and relieves tension and fatigue by stimulating circulation.

You can use a similar technique to relax *your* muscles. Stand with your feet about 18 inches apart, bend forward at your waist, and let your arms hang down relaxed. Then bend your knees a little and shift your weight from side to side so that your arms swing like a pendulum (or like an elephant's trunk). The rhythmical contraction and relaxation of your muscles will *force* relaxation of tense muscles and nerves. Many elderly persons get a similar effect by rocking in a rocking chair.

How Velma discharged her tensions

Velma H. was so tense that her back and neck muscles were actually inflamed from constant contraction. "I stay so tense and nervous," she complained, "that the slightest noise causes me to jump. My muscles ache constantly, and I cannot even sit down and relax. My doctor gives me pain pills and tranquilizers." I recommended the elephant swing for Velma. She did the exercise several times during the day—whenever she felt her tension building and her muscles tightening. Her tension was relieved immediately. And after a few weeks, her muscle soreness disappeared. "After doing that simple little exercise," she reported, "I can sit down and be completely relaxed. It's a wonderful treatment."

How to Break Tension by Relaxing Your Back Muscles and Loosening Your Spine

In my practice as a chiropractor, I've found that many aches and pains in nervous patients can be relieved by relaxing the muscles and joints of the back. In practically every form of tension, there is tightness in the muscles of the back and the neck. Conversely, when these muscles relax, the rest of the body relaxes. Complete relaxation quells nervous storms so that the organs of the body can function without the disturbing influence of agitated nerves. This is one reason why so many people feel that manipulation of the spine helps so many different ailments.

How to massage the back to relieve contracted and knotty muscles

You can get an effective back massage right in your own home. And with a few special instructions, any member of your family can loosen your vertebrae.

First wring out a few towels in hot water and apply them to the back to stimulate circulation and to aid relaxation. When the towels are removed, apply some type of oil (vegetable oil will be fine) to the muscles of the back. Masseurs often mix alcohol and mineral oil so that when the alcohol evaporates it will leave a thin layer of oil on the skin.

To massage the back, just cup your thumb and forefinger over the ridges of muscles that run up and down both sides of the spine and then rub from bottom to top in short, overlapping strokes. Move both hands together until you have covered the entire length of the spine. When you reach the neck, stroke the big muscles that run from the tip of the shoulder to the base of the skull.

Don't ever hack or thump the back. All that's necessary for complete relaxation is a gentle but firm kneading. *You can get just as much tension relief from a back massage as from an overall body massage.* If you do attempt to massage the entire body, always rub toward the heart in order to aid the circulation of venous blood. Remember that slow, gentle stroking *relaxes* muscles, while fast, vigorous stroking *stimulates* muscles.

When the massage is completed, the oil can be removed with rubbing alcohol. Simply wiping the skin with a moist cloth will remove most of the oil. When the skin is dry or chapped, it's best to leave a little oil on the skin.

How to loosen the vertebrae for total relaxation

For a deeper, more relaxing back treatment, you can follow back massage with an adjustment of the vertebrae between the shoulder blades. Professional manipulators charge several dollars to perform this simple adjustment. You can do it safely in your own home and as often as you like. *This manipulation is one of the big bonuses of this book, so don't fail to try it.*

The sofa-cushion adjustment technique: Place three sofa cushions end-to-end on the floor and instruct the "patient" to lie face down on the cushions with his chin hanging over the edge of the first cushion and both forearms resting on the floor alongside the cushion. Straddle the patient (with your knees on the floor) and place your hands palms-down in the center of his back so that your thumbs are parallel and about one inch apart. Rotate your wrists inward a little so that all of the pressure is on the thick muscle that lies on the thumb side of your palms. Press downward and slightly headward until the skin is pulled tight and the spine is pressed down. *Then, with a short, quick movement, thrust about one inch further.* (See Figure 2.)

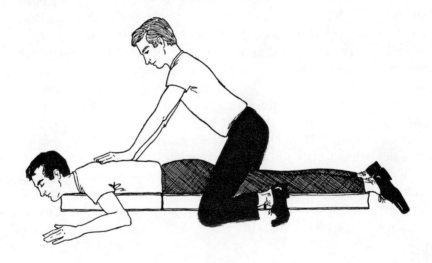

Drawing by Bibiana Neal

Figure 2. Sofa cushion technique position for relaxation.

For relaxation purposes, a single thrust between the shoulder blades will be adequate. You may, however, thrust over all the vertebrae that have ribs attached to them. Just begin at the bottom of the neck and work down over the next 12 vertebrae.

Before making each thrust, instruct the patient to take a deep breath so that he can exhale. Make the thrust at the end of the exhalation. It's important that the patient's glottis (throat) be left open so that no air is trapped in the lungs during the thrust. If the patient succeeds in relaxing during the adjustment, and can avoid holding his breath, there may be several audible *clicks* when the vertebrae move. This will be followed by an immediate sense of relief from tension.

This manipulation may also be used to relieve spasm and "catches" in the upper back. A bus driver, for example, who suffers from pain and muscle spasm between his shoulder blades at the end of a long trip reports that his wife can always relieve his discomfort with the sofa-cushion adjustment. I've recommended this home adjustment for many of my patients who have postural back pain, and all report good results.

Warning: Do not attempt to adjust the neck or the lower spine. Work only over the portion of the spine between the shoulder blades. If the back has been previously massaged with oil, remove the oil with rubbing alcohol and then dry the skin with a paper towel *before* making the adjustment.

How to Stretch Out Tension by Stretching Your Back

You can stretch tight back muscles and loosen spinal vertebrae by hanging on a ladder. Prop a ladder up against a wall at a steep angle. Step up on the bottom rung and then turn over on your back and reach up and grasp a rung at arm's length. Remove your feet from the bottom rung and hang relaxed for several seconds. The pressure of the rungs against your upper back while your muscles are being stretched will reverse the sagging strain caused by the pull of gravity.

Lying on a slant board with your feet anchored at the high end of the board will give your spine a relaxing stretch.

Relax with a Warm Tub Bath

A warm tub bath is usually very effective in relaxing muscles and inducing sleep. It's important, however, that the temperature of the water not be any higher than 98 degrees Fahrenheit. Water that is too hot (or too cold) will be stimulating rather than relaxing. Try to maintain a temperature of 94 to 98 degrees by adjusting the inflow and outflow so that there is rapid circulation of water.

A glass of warm milk following a warm bath will relax stomach muscles and provide soothing calcium for your nerves.

How to "Knock Out" Tension with a Neutral Wet-Sheet Pack

A neutral wet-sheet pack applied at home is a sure way to relieve tension and calm nerves. Most people find this treatment so restful that they actually fall asleep during its application. The patient is simply wrapped first in a cool, moist sheet and then in a couple of dry, woolen blankets to prevent rapid evaporation of the moisture. The body then warms itself with its own blood flow. If the correct procedure is followed, a neutral or slightly warm temperature can be maintained for total relaxation.

Four simple steps for using the wet-sheet pack effectively

Step 1. Cover your mattress with a plastic or rubber sheet and two woolen blankets. Wring out a smooth linen sheet (until it's nearly dry) in water that has a temperature of 60 to 70 degrees Fahrenheit. Lay the moist sheet over the blankets.

Step 2. Lie down on the sheet and lift your arms while half of the sheet is being wrapped around your body from your armpits to your feet.

Step 3. Then lower your arms so that the remaining half of the sheet can be wrapped around your entire body. This will cover your arms in such a way that there is no contact between bare skin surfaces. (The lower half of your body should be wrapped loosely so that the loose sheet can be pressed down between your legs.)

Step 4. Next, have someone cover you with the woolen blankets by folding them over—one at a time—so that they can be overlapped and tucked under your body for a close fit.

The wet sheet will feel cold at first. But after a few minutes you'll begin to experience a relaxing warmth. If your feet feel cold, have someone place a hot water bottle against the bottom of your feet. An extra blanket or two laid over your body will hasten warming.

For a good sedative effect, it's important that you do not get too warm. There should be a constant neutral temperature of about 94 degrees, which is slightly warmer than skin temperature. Remember that the neutral wet-sheet pack is not a heat treatment. When you begin to get more than warm, start peeling back the blankets until you're satisfied that the temperature will remain constantly neutral.

Make sure that the remaining blankets are sufficiently sealed around your neck and your feet to prevent the circulation of air around the sheet. Otherwise, you'll get cold rather than warm. One-half hour to one hour in the pack should be sufficient to relax you to the point of sleep. When the pack is removed, rub your body with a cold wash cloth for a tonic effect.

"Every doctor I have ever been to has told me to relax and quit worrying," said John C., a victim of hypertension and arthritis. "You're the first doctor to recommend something that I can actually do to relieve my tension. Since I've started using the wet-sheet pack, I can actually put myself to sleep. My blood pressure has dropped considerably and my arthritis is much better."

Many different illnesses caused by stress can be relieved with a relaxing neutral wet-sheet pack. It won't cost you a cent, and it may save you thousands of dollars in medical expenses.

Note: Elderly persons and heart patients who do not react beneficially to a neutral wet-sheet pack, or who are chilled by the moist sheet, should stick with the warm tub bath for relaxation.

How to Combat Stress with Diet

A body under stress needs more nutrients than does a relaxed, sedentary body, just as a racing engine needs more gas. Experiments with animals have revealed that any animal quickly becomes deficient in *all* the essential nutrients when it is subjected to unrelenting stress. The same is probably also true of humans. So try to make sure that you eat plenty of vitamin-rich natural foods every day. But don't overeat! An overstuffed stomach, like an overweight body, places damaging stress on the organs of the body.

When stress seems to be getting the best of you take some additional Vitamin C to protect your tissues, along with a little extra Vitamin B for your nervous system. Both of these vitamins, particularly Vitamin C, are rapidly depleted by nervous tension. Since all the B vitamins work together, I usually recommend Vitamin B complex rather than a single B vitamin. Pantothenic acid, which is a B vitamin, is believed to be especially effective in combating stress.

Certain fresh, natural foods, such as liver, wheat germ, and green leafy vegetables, contain "anti-stress factors" that seem to aid in overcoming the effects of stress.

Iodine is important
in controlling nerves

Make sure that your diet contains plenty of iodine-rich foods. Iodine is essential for the function of the thyroid gland, which secretes a hormone that influences the nervous system. When there is a deficiency of iodine, a malfunction in the thyroid gland may cause all sorts of nervous symptoms that will make it impossible for you to relax or sleep well.

Seafoods are the best sources of iodine. If you don't like fish, you can get adequate iodine from kelp, or dried seaweed. In areas where the soil is rich in iodine, the vegetables will contain iodine. Whenever possible, however, you should try to get your iodine from seafood.

How to Handle Bell's Palsy at Home

When the face is exposed to chilling wind or water, swelling of soft tissues sometimes pinches a facial nerve that passes through a small bony opening. This results in a temporary paralysis on one side of the face. If this happens to you, don't panic. The paralysis usually disappears after a month or two.

Simple moist heat applications applied to the affected side of the face will speed recovery. And plenty of Vitamin B complex will help rebuild the damaged nerve. You can maintain muscle tone by massaging the muscles of the face in an upward direction for about five minutes several times a day. If you like, you may also tape the face with Scotch tape to hold up sagging facial muscles.

If you're unable to blink your eye on the paralyzed side, you may have to wear a patch over the eye to keep the eye closed and to prevent drying and irritation of the eye ball. A drop of mineral oil in the eye each morning and night will protect sensitive membranes. Be sure to protect your face from extreme temperatures.

Simple Measures for Neuritis and Neuralgia

Inflammation of the nerves causes generalized aches and pains that are usually accompanied by a variety of strange sensations. Patients often say, for example, that it feels as if hot or cold water is being poured over a portion of their body, or that bugs are crawling over their skin.

Moderately warm moist heat applications or a warm bath, with plenty of Vitamin B complex, should help. Wheat germ and brewer's yeast are rich sources of all the B vitamins.

For lasting warmth and glow from a tub bath, add one to two tablespoons of table mustard to each gallon of water—at a temperature of about 80 to 90 degrees. Soak for about 20 minutes.

How to Be the Master of Your Own Mind

No matter what measures you take to eliminate stress or to control the effects of stress, you must learn to condition your mind so that you are in full control of your emotions. Otherwise, even the most minor form of stress can balloon into a dangerous form of stress. Some people, for example, experience more stress when they are Christmas shopping than some executives do who close million dollar deals. *Don't let your own mind create unnecessary stress,* and don't let your day make a slave out of you.

How to relieve your hostilities
with "war games"

If you're seething with anger and resentment after a day of pressure or harassment, you should do something *physical* to work off the excess adrenalin and to divert your mind. Any type of exercise, such as swimming, jogging, or punching a bag, is great for relieving tension. You can at least get out and rake the yards, dig in your garden, or hammer a few nails. I know one man who relieves his tension and his hostilities by yelling as loud as he can during private karate practice. He simply hacks and kicks imaginary enemies until he is calm and relaxed. "It sure is a lot easier on my wife and family if I can work off my tension *before* I get home," he said. "Until I started taking karate, I almost broke up my marriage with temper tantrums."

How to talk away your tensions

Some people can "talk out" their anger and their frustrations. So if some member of your family attempts to express a grievance, be sure to lend a friendly ear. Your patience and your willingness to listen may help prevent illness or hostility that could place hardship on the whole family.

Simply "speaking your piece" when you are faced with injustice or when someone or something is bothering you will very often vent dangerous tension. You must be careful, however, not to hurt someone's feelings by speaking too harshly. If you must express hostility, do it in sports or in vigorous physical exercise.

Don't create stress
with unnecessary responsibilities

Many people create unbearable stress by loading themselves with impossible obligations. Spending too much money for homes and cars, for example, so that finances are strained to the breaking point, is a common cause of damaging stress. If you spend more money than you earn, with nothing in reserve, you can't help worrying about losing everything in an unforeseen emergency.

Set sensible goals

It's good to be ambitious, but don't set your goals too high. "Fight always for the highest attainable aim, but don't put up resistance in vain." Make sure that your goals in life are within your capability and that they are obtainable.

Plan each day so that you'll have enough time to accomplish all the things you want to do. But don't try to do too much. If you don't have enough time to eat, sleep, exercise, make love, and do all the other things that are essential for health and happiness, a combination of stress and poor health will surely kill you.

Summary

1. Drugless methods designed to relieve tension will also relieve many symptoms and diseases that are caused by stress.
2. Techniques that relax your muscles, as in the elephant swing and the breathe-and-flop exercise, will relax nerves as well as relieve stress.
3. Massaging the muscles of the back from bottom to top will relieve tension just as effectively as an overall body massage.
4. A simple adjustment of the vertebrae between the shoulder blades, which can be performed on three sofa cushions, will break the cycle of tension between nerves and muscles.
5. A warm tub bath with water about 98 degrees Fahrenheit is great for relaxing tense muscles and inducing sleep.
6. A neutral wet-sheet pack, in which a temperature slightly higher than skin temperature is maintained for half an hour or so, has potent sedative effects that will relieve symptoms of stress.
7. During periods of stress, increase your intake of vitamin-rich natural foods and take a supplement containing Vitamins B and C.
8. Simple moist heat applications, Vitamin B complex, and facial massage will speed recovery from the paralysis caused by Bell's palsy.
9. Neuritis and neuralgia respond to moist heat and Vitamin B complex.
10. Don't create stress by striving for unattainable goals, by going deeply into debt, or by trying to crowd too much activity into each day.

4

How to Relieve Daily Aches
and Pains with Good Body
Mechanics and Proper Foot Care

In addition to causing many aches and pains, bad body mechanics can cause all sorts of disease. Poor posture, for example, can squeeze the life out of internal organs by compressing the chest and the abdomen. Irritation of spinal nerves causes radiating pains that reach into every portion of the body.

The condition of your feet can have a lot to do with your aches and pains. When your arches fall, for example, rotation of your legs and your pelvis places a strain on your spine that is transmitted all the way to the back of your neck! Everyone knows that when your feet suffer you suffer all over—physically and emotionally.

So remember that *everything you do to relieve pain by improving your posture and correcting your foot troubles will help you overcome a great variety of common and not-so-common ailments.* This chapter will show you how to get this health bonus. And the portion of this chapter dealing with foot problems will describe home-treatment methods that will provide welcome relief for suffering feet.

How You Can Relieve Pain and Cure Disease with Good Posture

When the spine sags, a great many things happen: an exaggerated neck curve causes headache, neck pain, and arm pain (brachial neuritis). A sagging shoulder girdle causes upper back and shoulder pain. A drooping chest squeezes the heart and lungs and interferes with the action of the diaphragm, causing shortness of breath and poor circulation. Pinched nerves cause chest pain (intercostal neuralgia) that resembles heart pain. The movement of shoulder blades over a rounded back grinds against the ribs and causes scapulothoracic bursitis. A relaxed abdominal wall allows organs to fall and press against each other, obstructing the flow of blood. This can contribute to the development of almost any type of organic disease. Constipation, painful menstruation, and varicose veins commonly result from postural pot belly. Circulatory interference in the abdomen places considerable strain on the heart and raises blood pressure.

And that's not all. Shifting of the center of balance in the lower back strains muscles and ligaments, jams spinal joints together, and causes leg pain (sciatic neuritis) by pinching nerves. Arthritis develops in irritated joints. Overworked muscles that are straining against the pull of gravity become inflamed and spastic. All this leads to fatigue and lowered resistance that makes you more susceptible to disease and infection.

Obviously, one of the first things you should do to relieve your aches and pains and improve your health is to correct your posture. Many vague symptoms will disappear as if by magic when your joints are properly aligned.

How posture was the key to Marilyn's aches and pains

Marilyn R., a dental assistant, had complained of backache and a variety of aches and pains for several years. Recurring abdominal and chest pains had defied diagnosis in numerous visits to dozens of doctors. "I have these shooting pains," she said, "that have been falsely diagnosed as heart trouble, gall stones, and renal colic. Nothing I do seems to help."

One look at Marilyn's posture gave me a clue to the origin of her pains. Her spine slumped so badly that a grotesquely rounded back was made even more grotesque by a protruding, relaxed abdominal wall. I instructed her in the basic rules of good posture and asked her to call me back in a couple of months. I was pleased to hear that her pains disappeared as her posture improved.

**Four simple rules for pain-free
standing posture**

Having good posture for good body mechanics does not mean
that you have to walk around as rigid as a toy soldier. With truly
good posture, you should be able to move about freely and easily
with a minimum amount of strain or fatigue. Don't worry about
comparing your posture with that of other people. The best
posture for you may be unique. Just follow these simple rules, and
then be guided by the results.

Rule 1. When you are standing or walking, *stand tall* so that you
maintain your maximum height. Be careful not to exaggerate your
efforts to stand properly. If you do, your muscles will quickly
"give out" and your body will sag back into its same old posture.

Rule 2. Lift your chest just a little. Slight elevation of your ribs
will lift your diaphragm and relieve compression on your abdominal organs as well as allow deeper breathing. An occasional deep
inspiration high into your chest will aid venous blood flow by
exerting a suction effect on the big vein that returns blood to your
heart.

Rule 3. Hold your abdomen in just enough to keep your
abdominal wall from sagging. Practice drawing in your abdomen
every chance you get. *The ability to control your abdominal
muscles is an important key to good body mechanics.* Remember
that a flat abdomen provides a muscular corset that helps hold
every organ in its proper position.

Rule 4. If you have a "sway back," tuck your hips under just
enough to take the excessive arch out of your lower back.
Otherwise, you'll develop a relaxed abdominal wall and a pot belly
along with backache—and this is a combination that can cause a
great deal of misery.

Once good posture becomes a habit, you won't even be aware
of your efforts to maintain the posture. Bad posture, on the other
hand, greatly overworks muscles and causes painful fatigue.

Proper Sitting Posture Relieves Back and Leg Pain
and Aids Recovery from Organic Disease

Good sitting posture is just as important as good standing
posture. Actually, allowing your chest and spine to slump while

sitting places *more* pressure on your back and your internal organs than would occur while standing improperly.

Two rules for healthful stress-free sitting posture

Rule 1. Sit erect (in a straight-back chair whenever possible) with a slight arch in your lower back. Scoot back in the chair so that your buttocks touch the chair back. Otherwise, attempts to lean back will round out your lower back and place damaging pressure on your tailbone.

A special low-back support. If you find it difficult to sit erect, especially when driving, place a thin pad in the hollow of your lower back. A small towel folded over three or four times should be fine. For people who travel a great deal, I sometimes recommend that they wrap a pocket-size paperback book in a hand towel and then stitch the edges of the towel to make a permanent pad. If you like, you can use a couple of cords to suspend the pad on the back of the seat so that it will hang in just the right place to fit into the arch of your lower back.

How a traveling salesman eased his aching back

Monte W. was a traveling salesman who had been suffering from backache for several years. "My back stays sore and stiff all the time," he complained. "And sometimes after a long trip I can hardly get in and out of my car." I personally helped Monte suspend a small supporting cushion on the back of his car seat. He began to feel better after the first day. When I saw him a month later, his back trouble was nearly gone. "I never would have thought that such a simple measure would do so much good," he reported with amazement.

Rule 2. Select a chair that's just high enough to place your thighs and legs at right angles to each other without excessive pressure between the back of your thighs and the front edge of the chair seat. Both feet should be parallel and flat on the floor.

If you must sit long hours in your employment, it's especially important that you have good sitting posture. A chair that's too high can cause leg pain and muscle paralysis by compressing nerves and blood vessels behind the knee.

Reverse Postural Strain and Relieve Compression
Pain with a Slant Board

If you suffer from pain and fatigue caused by bad posture, there is a single relaxing posture that you can assume to relieve the symptoms and reverse the strain.

Visit the lumber yard and purchase a smooth, wide board that's thick enough to support your weight without sagging and long enough to reach beyond your head and your feet. Encircle one end of the board with an old belt or a strap and secure it so that it hangs loosely on one side of the board. Prop the strapped end of the board up on a chair or a table top, anchor your feet under the strap, and then lie on the board relaxed. The upside-down position will aid venous circulation, stretch your spine, and reverse the pull on sagging abdominal organs. The steeper the incline, the greater the pull. A few minutes on the board will completely relieve pains caused by pressure on joints, nerves, and organs.

A thin cushion under your upper back while you are lying on the board will force correction of a slumping, rounded back. Lower-back discomfort can be relieved by placing a thin pillow under both knees.

How to Balance Your Body and Relieve Muscle and
Joint Pains with Good Foot Posture

No matter how much of an effort you make to maintain good standing posture, you won't succeed if you have bad foot posture. Your feet form the foundation for your entire body. When they are out of balance, the rest of your body is out of balance.

The most common fault in bad foot posture is a rolling in of both ankles. This can result from fallen arches, tight ankle tendons, or a slew-footed stance. When the ankles do roll toward each other, the lower legs rotate, forcing the knees to rotate toward each other. This produces sway back by tilting the pelvis forward. Every portion of the body must make certain changes to accommodate the unbalanced feet. I've seen many patients with *foot pain, knee pain, hip pain, backache, headache, muscle spasm, shoulder pain, and other symptoms* that could be traced to bad feet.

Fallen arches need support

A bank guard who spent several hours a day on his feet suffered constantly with arch and ankle pains. At the end of the day, he also complained of backache and headache. When he employed simple measures to lift his arches and correct his slew-footed stance, his aches and pains disappeared—simply because realigning his feet had relieved the tension in certain spinal muscles.

If you have fallen arches or flat feet, get a good pair of shoes and fit them with arch supports. A ready-made, leather-covered rubber support that's sold in many shoe stores and drug stores may be adequate. If not, a podiatrist can build a pair that will fit your feet.

Point your toes straight ahead to relieve ankle and arch pain

When you stand or walk, you should point your toes nearly straight ahead. You should lift your arches slightly so that most of your weight is supported on the outside edges of the soles of your feet. This will activate the muscular sling that supports the arch of your feet. Even when you're wearing shoes with arch supports, you should make a conscious effort to lift your arches a little.

A special heel for weak feet

If you're overweight and you feel that there is excessive strain on your arches, a *Thomas heel* will help your feet support your weight. This is a special heel that's longer and thicker on one side. You can get one in any shoe shop.

How to use sole wedges to correct slew foot

If you habitually walk slew-footed and you find it difficult to walk with your toes pointed straight ahead, a one-eighth-inch tapered wedge inserted between the inner and outer soles on the

inside edge of the soles of your shoes might help. The wedge will
lift the inside portion of your shoes and turn your feet inward. If
your shoe repairman is not familar with the use of sole wedges, try
an orthopedic shoe shop.

Note: If you're pigeon-toed, the wedge should be placed on the
outside edge of the shoe sole.

Give your suffering feet a break!

A normal foot should be more than strong enough to support
your weight, even when you are barefoot. In fact, failure to go
without shoes occasionally will actually weaken your feet. So if
your feet aren't already broken down, kick off your shoes every
chance you get and walk around in your bare feet.

How to Relieve Foot Pain with Special Pads and Home Treatment

Jackie C. had a severe pain between the second and third toes
on her right foot when she stood and walked. She tried several
different pairs of shoes in a vain effort to relieve her pain. She also
visited several doctors, one of whom prescribed two weeks of
physical therapy. Nothing helped. All she needed to relieve her
pain was a small shoe pad that could be purchased in any shoe
store for less than one dollar!

A metatarsal pad relieves pain
in the front of the foot

If you have pain in the front part of your foot (caused by a
callus, a plantar wart, or by pinching and jamming of nerves and
bones), a metatarsal pad placed under the front of the foot or
just behind the painful spot may shift weight bearing enough to
relieve the pain. A painful callus on the ball of the foot can
be relieved by placing the metatarsal pad *behind* the callus.

Most shoe stores and drug stores sell these small circular pads
(some in combination with arch supports). An experienced shoe
salesman may be able to help you place the pad in the right spot in

your shoe. It is sometimes necessary to tape the pad to the bottom of the foot to maintain proper positioning.

A metatarsal bar is sometimes best

If a metatarsal pad does not seem to help, or if the pain or callus is near the outside edges of the foot, a metatarsal bar placed just behind the balls of the foot may help. This is simply a long, thin bar that spans the width of the foot.

A felt bar may be placed inside the shoe, or a leather bar may be attached to the outside of the shoe (under the sole). The outside bar is usually the most effective. You can buy ready-made inside-metatarsal bars in many drug stores. Some shoe shops, or any orthopedic shop, can attach an outside-metatarsal bar to your shoe.

Females who have foot troubles should wear low-heeled, oxford-type shoes to accommodate pads, bars, and other alterations. The use of pads of any type with high-heeled shoes may only increase the pain.

Note: If you do a lot of walking or jogging, a persistent, stubborn pain in the front part of your foot may be the result of a "spontaneous" fracture called a "march fracture." An X-ray examination of the foot will usually reveal the presence of such a fracture. The fracture will usually heal with rest and the support of a good, properly fitted leather shoe.

How to Relieve the Pain of a Heel Spur

A "heel spur" means just what it implies. A sharp, bony projection on the bottom of the heel bone jabs the overlying soft tissues when pressure is placed on the heel. Anything you can do to relieve this pressure when you stand and walk will help relieve the pain.

How to alter the heel of your shoe

Shoes should, of course, have *rubber* heels to cushion the impact of walking. When the spur is not too large, a sponge rubber pad placed inside the shoe, or a piece of felt with a hole cut in it to relieve pressure on the painful spot, may help. In more severe cases, it may be necessary to gouge a hole into the heel of the shoe (from the inside) and then fill the cavity with sponge rubber so that there is no direct pressure on the spur. Try it first on an old pair of shoes so that you can decide exactly where and how large the hole should be before you start gouging into your best pair of shoes. An arch support may also help relieve weight on a painful heel.

A female sales clerk who limped into my office with *three* spurs on the same heel obtained complete relief by gouging out the inside of her shoe. When I saw her last, she was darting from store to store in a shopping spree. A man who had suffered for several years with a painful heel spur obtained relief by reducing his body weight and wearing shoes with rubber heels.

What to Do About Corns, Calluses, and Bunions

Most corns and calluses on the feet are caused by tight or improperly fitted shoes that rub the skin and squeeze the feet. Constant, unrelieved pressure over bony areas can cause corns by interfering with the circulation of blood. If your shoes are too tight and you cannot afford to buy another pair, it would be better to slit the leather to relieve pressure over the trouble spots than to allow your feet to suffer.

When you walk or jog a long distance, wearing two pairs of thin socks will protect your feet from blisters by reducing friction between your feet and your shoes. A little Vaseline petroleum jelly between your toes will prevent irritating contact between moist skin surfaces.

You'll learn later in this chapter how to protect your feet with properly fitted shoes. In the meantime, if you already have corns and calluses, there is a great deal that you can do to ease your discomfort.

Trim corns carefully

Corns and calluses that have been softened by soaking the feet in hot, soapy water can be trimmed with a sharp knife or a dull, used razor blade that has been sterilized with alcohol. You must be *very careful,* however, not to cut too deeply, lest you develop a painful infection. Always trim toward the center of the corn. Just circle the corn from its outer edge and keep the blade parallel to the skin. Stop if you feel pain or see blood. Removal of too much tissue can produce a painful scar.

Just to be safe, *cut away only a small part of the top portion of the corn and then finish the job with an emery board.* This way, you won't be able to cut too deeply. You can periodically file away a new build-up of tissue.

Warning: If you have diabetes, let a podiatrist trim your corns. Cutting too deeply could lead to a serious infection. Poor circulation caused by hardened arteries can delay healing.

How to prevent painful irritation of corns

If your shoes aren't too tight, sponge rubber pads may be taped over freshly trimmed corns and calluses to prevent irritation of sensitive tissue.

When corns begin to develop between the toes, a little Vaseline petroleum jelly or lamb's wool between the offending toes will help by reducing friction and preventing contact between soggy skin surfaces.

You should, of course, go without shoes as much as possible. During the summer, when I am not in my office, I wear rubber sandals that cover only the soles of my feet. You can buy such a sandal in any dime store for only a few cents. You probably shouldn't walk on the ground in your bare feet, since you might pick up parasites and other infections.

Fight corns with Vitamin A

Vitamin A is sometimes recommended to speed recovery from severe or resistant corns and calluses. As much as 100,000 units daily for a month or longer have been prescribed by some physicians. It's important to remember, however, that large doses of Vitamin A over a long period of time can have toxic effects. So you must be cautious about taking this vitamin. The minimum daily requirement for Vitamin A calls for 5,000 units, but you may safely take 25,000 units daily for a few months at a time. Always buy the natural Vitamin A—or eat plenty of green and yellow fruits and vegetables and take a supplement containing fish liver oil.

How to stretch away your bunions

Bunions, which are often associated with partial dislocation of the big toe, are most often caused by shoes that squeeze the toes. A build-up of bone and callus, or enlargement of the bursa at the base of the big toe, may make full correction impossible—but. there's plenty that you can do.

Always select shoes that have a straight inner margin that will conform to the inside border of your foot. This will prevent bunion-causing pressure against the big toe.

In the early stages of bunion development, a pad placed between the first two toes will help keep the big toe in line. *Regular stretching of the big toe in a corrective direction will prevent shortening of ligaments.* If you wear shoes with pointed toes, you should stretch and pull your big toe away from the second toe every time you pull off your shoes.

How to Stop Ingrowing Toenails

Toenails, especially the nail of the big toe, should be cut squarely across so that the corners of the nail project beyond the skin. When the corners of a nail are trimmed or rounded, they tend to grow into the flesh. Shoes that crowd the toes together will painfully aggravate an ingrown toenail.

At the first signs of an ingrown toenail, pack Vaseline-soaked gauze or a wisp of cotton under the corners of the nail and let it grow out so that it can be cut straight across. Wear a wide-toed shoe that won't squeeze your toes together or place any pressure on your toenails. A stretch sock, or a sock that is too tight, will put painful pressure on an ingrown nail.

Onychogryposis—The Thick Toenail

A big-toe nail will occasionally become thick, rough, and dark following injury or interference with circulation. The treatment is simple. Just remove all pressure from the nail, file the nail down, and use foot baths to improve the circulation of blood.

This condition is common among women who wear high-heeled shoes that have pointed toes—and it snags many a nylon stocking!

How to Get Rid of Athlete's Foot

Having athlete's foot has nothing to do with being an athlete. People from all walks of life suffer from this aggravating, itchy affliction. When it's allowed to continue unchecked, it can lead to infection, swelling, and crippling disability. A hospital janitor, for example, had such a severe case of athlete's foot that he could not even walk! His feet were so swollen and cracked that he was unable to wear his shoes. The medication his doctor had prescribed did not seem to help. When he used my simple home-care methods, however, his feet quickly healed.

Home treatment for athlete's foot

Athlete's foot is caused by a fungus that thrives on wet, soggy skin. The best treatment, therefore, is to *keep the feet as dry as possible.*

After bathing, dry your feet and toes thoroughly and then sprinkle them with medicated powder before putting on your socks. Lamb's wool may be placed between the toes to prevent contact between raw, moist skin surfaces. Use thick, white cotton socks that will absorb moisture and allow the circulation of air. During the summer, wear perforated shoes or sandals for maximum ventilation. *Expose your feet to sun and air as often as possible.* Generous doses of Vitamins A and C will fight off infection.

How to Detect and Control Gout in Your Body

If your big toe, ankle, or heel ever becomes swollen, hot, red, and exquisitely painful for no apparent reason, don't take it for granted that your shoes are at fault. *You may have gout.* This is a condition in which your body is unable to eliminate the uric acid by-products of protein metabolism, allowing them to accumulate in the tissue around certain joints.

Harry J., a building contractor, suffered from recurring attacks of gout in his wrist and his big toe. Since the pain always subsided after a few days, he didn't bother to see his doctor. So he never did find out what was wrong. Eventually, however, the uric acid deposits in his big toe became so great that a draining abscess developed. Had Harry known that the heavy protein diet he was on was responsible for the progress of the disease, he could have controlled it with dietary measures. (Not everyone who eats foods containing uric acid or purines will develop gout. This happens only in people who develop metabolic problems involving elimination of body wastes.)

A low-purine diet for
controlling uric acid

A test measuring the amount of uric acid in your blood will tell you whether you have gout or not. If you do, you'll have to restrict your intake of protein foods that are rich in purines or uric acid.

Here are some high-purine foods you must avoid: sweetbreads (animal pancreas or thymus), sardines, anchovies, kidney, liver, brain, meat, meat extracts, gravies, fish, game, fowl, beans, lentils, spices, condiments, and alcoholic beverages.

You can get adequate purine-free protein from nuts, seeds, skim milk, eggs, cheese, cottage cheese, gelatin, and protein supplements. Since whole grain wheat contains a moderate amount of purine, try to eat corn bread rather than wheat bread. Whole grain cereals can be replaced by grits or cream of wheat. Eat plenty of fruits and vegetables and drink plenty of liquids to aid your kidneys in eliminating uric acid, otherwise kidney stones may form. Fruit and vegetable juice will help alkalinize your blood and urine.

Cutting down on the purines in your diet and drinking about three quarts of liquids daily will literally wash the uric acid deposits out of your joints.

Shoes that are too tight tend to trigger attacks of gout in the feet of persons who have the disease. So make sure that your shoes are properly fitted.

How to make a tent
or cradle for your feet

When the big toe is undergoing a gouty attack, the weight of a bed sheet can cause agonizing pain. You can construct a light, wooden frame to place over your foot so that the bed covers won't rest against the painful toe. Or you can use an umbrella or a small chair to make a tent over your foot. When you get back on your feet, you may find it necessary to cut the toe out of the shoe on the affected side in order to wear shoes and get back to work. (See Figure 3.)

How to ease pain
with rest and compresses

An acutely painful attack of gout can often be relieved with a cold compress. If that doesn't seem to help, try a hot compress, applied every two or three hours. If necessary, your doctor can prescribe special drugs to relieve the pain temporarily and dissolve solid uric acid deposits contributing to the pain.

The Pain May Be Morton's Toe!

Carolee was being dined in an exclusive restaurant when she suddenly jerked off her shoe and started manipulating her foot. The scene would have been quite funny if it had not been so obvious that she was in severe pain. The expression of agony left after a few seconds, however, and she made a red-faced apology

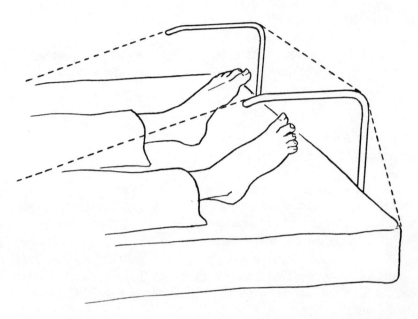

Drawing by Bibiana Neal

Figure 3. Details of a tent for the feet in bed.

while she replaced her shoe. "I've had the pain before," she said. "My doctor calls it Morton's toe."

If you're ever suddenly stricken with a sudden, sharp, burning pain that seems to be limited to a single toe other than the big toe, you might also be suffering from Morton's toe. This is a condition in which the bones of the feet pinch a nerve at the base of the affected toe.

How to relieve pain
by manipulating your foot

Manipulating your bare foot with both hands will very often relieve pain caused by pinched nerves and jammed bones. Just twist, pull, and bend the front part of the foot until the pain goes away. An arch support or a metatarsal pad may help to prevent recurrences of the pain.

In the early stages of Morton's toe, before the pain begins, there may be a burning sensation at the base of the toe, along with a little numbness. This may be a warning that your shoes are too tight.

How to Relieve Foot Pain with Properly Fitted Shoes

A properly fitted shoe is essential for complete relief from foot pain. People who walk or stand a great deal should always select a good leather shoe that has fairly thick soles, low heels, and a rigid shank. (The shank is the portion of the shoe between the heel and the front sole.) The front of the shoe should be wide enough to accommodate your toes without squeezing them when you stand— and it should be one-quarter to one-half inch longer than your longest toe.

An important rule for fitting shoes

It's very important that the ball of the foot just behind the big toe rest exactly at the point where the inside margin of the sole begins to curve inward under the arch. If the shoe is too long and the base of the big toe is too far forward, the instep of the shoe will not fit the arch of your foot.

Be guided by the way you feel. If a shoe hurts or squeezes your foot, you know that the shoe is the wrong size. Remember that a shoe should conform to the shape of your foot. You should *never* force your foot to fit a shoe.

If you don't already have fallen arches, *don't buy shoes with built-in arch supports.* Unnecessary support will only weaken your arches. A normal, healthy arch is more than strong enough to support your body weight, even when you are barefoot.

What to do about painful heels

It's very important that the counter or heel portion of the shoe be properly fitted. If the counter does not conform to the shape of the back of your heel, or if it slides up and down on your heel when you walk, you might develop blisters, heel bursitis, a callus, periostitis (inflammation of heel bone), tendonitis, synovitis, or heel spurs. If the shoes you now have are too loose, a shoe store can fill the space behind your heel by gluing a felt pad to the inside of the shoe counter.

A soft rubber pad with a hole cut in its center can be taped over the heel to relieve pressure on a painful spot. Whenever possible, however, you should go without your customary shoes until a painful heel is completely healed and then buy a properly fitted pair of shoes. Rest, hot applications, massage, and contrast baths will relieve symptoms and speed recovery.

Note: Women who are accustomed to wearing high-heeled shoes should not suddenly switch to low heels. A gradual reduction of heel height will prevent painful stretching of tight ankle tendons.

Any Kind of Foot Trouble Can Benefit from a Contrast Bath

No matter what type of foot trouble you have, a contrast bath will help relieve the symptoms. Because of the distance of the feet from the heart and the interference of gravity, the circulation of blood in the feet is often very poor. Improving circulation by alternating hot and cold foot baths will relieve pain as well as speed recovery from foot troubles.

Foot bath technique

Get two deep tubs or buckets that will hold enough water to reach well up on your calves. Fill one container with hot water (100 to 110 degrees F.) and the other with cold water (50 to 65 degrees). Place both feet in the hot water for three to five minutes and then in the cold water for one to two minutes. Five, seven, or nine immersions may be made, beginning and ending with the hot water.

After you dry your feet with a towel, rub a little oil on your feet and then massage and manipulate each foot for a minute or two. Stretch all of your toes. Twist the front part of each foot from side to side in a circular motion.

Warning: If you have very bad circulation caused by hardened arteries, you should avoid extreme water temperatures. If leg pain results from a contrast bath, discontinue the treatment—or try milder temperatures.

Summary

1. Good standing and sitting posture is an effective remedy for a great variety of aches and pains.
2. Sole wedges and other measures designed to correct a slew-footed stance will relieve pain and tension that extends all the way from the ankles to the back of the neck.
3. Pain felt in the front part of your foot when you stand can very often be relieved with metatarsal pads placed inside your shoe or with metatarsal bars glued to the bottom of your shoe.
4. When a painful heel spur is not relieved by rubber heels and sponge rubber padding, it may be necessary to gouge out the inside of your shoe heel and fill it with sponge rubber.
5. Corns and calluses can be trimmed away or filed down, but they will recur if excessive pressures on the foot aren't removed.
6. Bunions and ingrown toenails are most often caused by narrow-toed shoes that squeeze the toes together.
7. The best remedy for athlete's foot is to keep the feet—especially between the toes—as dry as possible.
8. Gout and Morton's toe are two painful foot disorders that require special measures for permanent relief.
9. A properly fitted shoe is an absolute necessity in the care of foot disorders of all types.
10. A contrast foot bath, followed by massage and manipulation of the foot, will provide instant relief for tired and aching feet.

5

First Aid Nature's Way
for Bruises, Strains, Sprains,
and Muscle Injuries

No matter how healthy you are, you won't be able to avoid an occasional strain or sprain. When you do suffer such an injury, quick use of nature's remedies will assure a full and speedy recovery. This chapter will tell you everything you need to know to care for your muscle injuries at home—and you won't need any special facilities.

How to Speed Recovery from a Sprained Ankle

Tommy B. stepped in a hole and twisted his ankle. A friend advised him to put the ankle in hot water—which he did. The next morning, the injured ankle was red, swollen, and throbbing with pain. So he again immersed the ankle in hot water. A few days later, both the ankle and the foot were tremendously swollen with black and blue discoloration. It took Tommy many weeks to get over his injury. Had the ankle been properly treated (at home), his disability would have lasted only a few days.

How to use cold packs to reduce
bleeding and cut down on swelling

The next time you turn your ankle enough to cause pain, apply an ice pack to the ankle as soon as possible. You can make an effective ice pack by filling a plastic bag with crushed ice and then wrapping it in a moist towel. If the pack seems to be too cold, use a dry towel rather than a moist towel. Keep the injured ankle elevated while the pack is being applied. A cold pack may be used continuously as long as comfort permits—or at least 20 to 30 minutes every two hours for the first day or so.

When you don't have the materials you need to make a cold pack, you may simply immerse your foot in cold water or apply towels that have been wrung out in cold water. Water that has a temperature of 50 to 60 degrees Fahrenheit should be cold enough for immersion. Take your foot out of the water for a few minutes when the cold seems to cause aching. If you use compresses or cold towels, they should be changed frequently to maintain the effects of cold.

Cold treatment cuts down on bleeding and swelling by constricting blood vessels. It should be applied at least once every two hours. Otherwise, the blood vessels will react later by dilating, thus increasing the amount of bleeding.

Warning: Except in special cases requiring ice massage, which you'll learn about later in this chapter, you should never apply ice directly to the skin. Prolonged contact with ice can result in an "ice burn."

How to wrap an injured ankle with an elastic bandage

When an ice pack is applied infrequently during the day, it might be a good idea to wrap the ankle between treatments to prevent swelling. A two- or three-inch elastic bandage crisscrossed snugly around the ankle and heel and under the arch for several turns should suffice. Wrap the ankle immediately after each cold treatment and after elevating the foot. If you prefer, you can purchase a special sock-type bandage that can be slipped over the foot and around the ankle.

After 36 to 48 hours, apply heat

After 36 to 48 hours have passed, you may apply heat to a sprained ankle to speed healing. Continued use of cold would only delay healing by reducing the flow of blood. Properly applied moist heat will *increase* the circulation of blood by dilating blood vessels. Apply hot compresses or immerse the ankle in comfortably hot water (about 105 degrees) for 15 or 20 minutes at a time several times a day.

Note: Even if you use cold treatment for only a few minutes or a few hours the first day, you should still wait at least 36 hours before applying heat. If the application of heat before 48 hours have passed causes pain, you should go back to the use of cold packs and wait until the next day before trying heat again.

When in doubt about whether to use heat or cold on an injury, always use cold—and try the heat later.

After the third day, use a contrast bath

After three or four days have passed, a contrast bath will break down stubborn clots and flush out clogged blood vessels. Immerse the foot in comfortably hot water for about four minutes and then in comfortably cold water for about two minutes. Repeat the cycle several times, beginning and ending with hot water. The heat will dilate or open the blood vessels, while the cold will constrict or close them. This has a pumping effect that will literally force the flow of blood through the injured tissues. Use the contrast bath at least twice daily—once in the morning and once in the evening.

I once recommended the contrast bath to a race driver who hobbled into my office (on crutches) with a badly sprained ankle that was still stiff and swollen *after four weeks of rest.* Two days later, he entered a stock car race and won!

How flushing his veins helped Russell walk soon again

A construction worker who had broken his ankle in an industrial accident continued to suffer with a swollen, painful ankle long after the bones had healed. "I'm still not able to walk," said Russell P.,"but my doctor says that he just doesn't know what else to do."

I explained to Russell that perhaps the foot needed flushing out to open clogged blood vessels so that the circulation would not be obstructed. I recommended the contrast bath, which he used three times daily for a couple of weeks. The swelling started to subside after the first day! By the end of the first week, he was back at work. All of the swelling and tenderness had disappeared by the end of the second week.

The contrast bath is a simple, harmless, but *effective* treatment that can benefit *any* chronic joint injury.

How to control swelling with Vitamin C

If you bruise easily, or if minor strains or bruises seem to result in excessive swelling or discoloration, you should increase your intake of Vitamin C to strengthen blood vessels and tissue cells. A *natural* Vitamin C supplement contains rutin, bioflavonoids, and other factors that increase the effectiveness of Vitamin C. Citrus fruit is a good source of Vitamin C, but you should eat the whole fruit rather than squeeze it for juice. Most of the bioflavonoids, for example, are found in the pulp and peeling of the fruit. Even the white substance that separates the peeling from the fruit should be eaten.

An important rule: always rest injured ligaments

When a joint has been strained or sprained, the ligaments are usually injured. This means that you must *rest* the joint until the ligaments have had a chance to heal. You can't work off the pain of a sprained ankle. So don't try it. You can get all the exercise you need for a sprained ankle by bending your foot in all directions while it is submerged in hot water.

Roundabout massage of an injured joint

In the early stages of an ankle sprain, the use of a contrast bath will provide a "physiological massage" by exercising the blood vessels. After three or four days, however, light fingertip massage may be used *around* the injured tissues. Just "milk" the tissues around the painful area by stroking toward the knee. As the ankle heals and the tissues become less painful, you can begin to stroke over the injured area lightly with your fingertips.

Hints on Caring for the Elbow, Knee, and Other Joints

When you strain or twist a knee, elbow, or wrist, you should *observe the same basic rules outlined for the care of a sprained ankle.* Use cold packs during the first 24 hours or so, but wait 36 to 48 hours before using heat. There are, however, some special steps that may be taken in the care of elbow and knee injuries.

Quick cold for elbow injuries

Many athletes apply cold to an injured elbow by sliding a portion of an inner tube over the arm before immersing the elbow in a tub of water containing ice cubes or crushed ice. The rubber prevents direct contact with the ice and allows even distribution of the cold.

If you watch baseball on television, you've probably seen trainers rush out on the field and spray something on a player's freshly injured elbow. This is a special chemical spray that chills the joint to relieve pain and reduce swelling. A plain cold pack is more effective, however, when you have the time to use it at home.

Special wrapping for the knee

When the knee is badly strained, a four-inch elastic bandage wrapped diagonally above and below the knee—while the knee is slightly bent—will provide steadying support.

Take a couple of anchor turns around the leg just below the knee cap. Run the bandage up *behind* the knee and take a turn above the knee cap. Then run the bandage down behind the knee again. Continue the wrapping, overlapping the bandage a couple of inches on each turn, until the entire knee is covered. Be careful not to wrap the knee too tightly. Too much pressure might obstruct the circulation of blood. Remember that an elastic bandage tends to tighten after wrapping.

Note: With the exception of the knee and the ankle, which are joints that must support your weight when you stand and walk, it's best to avoid wrapping a joint whenever possible. Routine wrapping of every injured joint may only delay healing by interfering with circulation and causing stiffness.

How to Unlock a Locked Knee

If you have ever torn a cartilage in your knee, a loose fragment might someday work loose and lock your knee joint so that you cannot straighten your leg. If this ever happens to you, there are some simple manipulations that you can use to unlock the knee. For example, Clyde M., a 46-year-old carpenter who had suffered a knee injury in football 28 years ago, discovered that he could get the "catches" out of his knee by swinging his leg from side to side. "Before I learned to do it myself," he said, "I had to hobble to an orthopedist every time my knee locked."

Self-manipulation won't always work, but it's worth trying. Here's what I suggest to my patients who suffer from recurring knee locks:

1. First sit on a high table, dangle your legs, and then swing the affected leg from side to side. Relax the leg muscles as much as possible.
2. If the first manipulation doesn't work, try this: Lie on your back (on the floor) with the knee of the affected leg bent and the foot flat on the floor. Have some member of the family place one hand on each side of the knee and toss it back and forth as if it were a hot potato.
3. Finally, as a last resort, use manipulation: Lie on your back with the knee of the affected leg bent. Determine which side of the knee is the most painful. (There are two cartilages in the knee—one on each side.) Instruct your helper to stand facing the side of the knee that is *not* painful. He may then grasp the ankle with one hand and the knee with the other hand and gently press toward the painful side while he slowly straightens

your leg. Let the bent leg flop over as far as necessary to place tension on the knee ligaments. When the knee joint spreads open on the painful side, the cartilage may slip back into place so that the leg can straighten out. Stop the manipulation if you feel any pain.

A Home-Care Program for Muscle Injuries

Anytime you suffer a bruise, a "charley horse," or a muscle injury that is severe enough to cause immediate pain, you should apply a cold pack to reduce bleeding in the injured tissues. An ice bag wrapped in a moist or dry towel, applied at least half an hour every two hours during the first day, will be fine. If you are a very active person, however, and you want to continue to use the muscle as much as possible, you might want to use *ice massage*.

How a thigh muscle injury was easily handled for a golfer

An attorney, Kenneth B., who badly bruised his thigh when he fell from a ladder, was frantic at the thought of not being able to participate in a golf tournament the next day. "I've *got* to play tomorrow," he said with a note of desperation. "I've been looking forward to being in this tournament, and now I can hardly walk. What am I going to do?"

I recommended the ice massage treatment for Kenneth. "Use the ice several times today and again in the morning, and maybe you'll be able to play tomorrow." Two days later, Kenneth called to say that he did very well in the tournament. "That ice massage was great," he said. "I got along fine and had very little pain."

This new and revolutionary treatment for muscle injuries is called *cryotherapy*. All you need for it is a little ice from your refrigerator.

How to use cryotherapy in treating muscle injuries

Fill a paper cup with water and freeze it so that it will be ready for use when an injury occurs. You can run a little hot water over the outside of the cup for easy removal of the cylinder of ice.

Rub a little oil over the skin of the injured muscle for protection against the shock of sudden cold. Then rub the muscle with the widest side of the ice cylinder. Use long, slow strokes up and down the length of the muscle. Continue the stroking until the skin becomes numb to the cold. There may be considerable aching or "burning" at first, but the muscle should begin to feel numb after about ten minutes of massage.

Repeat the massage several times throughout the day. If you can do so without pain, contract the injured muscle several times after each massage. (Combining ice massage and exercise is called *cryokinetics.*)

If the injury is very severe and muscle contraction is painful, it might be a good idea to apply cold cloths or an ice pack off and on between applications of ice massage.

Note: It will be necessary to wear a glove or grip the ice with a cloth in order to protect the hand holding the ice. Some people freeze ice cream sticks in the water in order to make a handle for holding the ice.

Remember that cold applications should not be applied longer than 48 hours. Once the bleeding stops, healing is best stimulated by moist heat applications.

How to work the "knots" out of injured muscles

Unlike ligament injuries, in which the injured joint must be rested until healing has occured, *injured muscles should be exercised as soon as possible.* When an injured muscle is rested too long, the escaped blood forms a knotty deposit that interferes with the movement of muscle fibers. If the deposit collects calcium (which may form bone), a permanent lump in the muscle may lead to frequent recurrences of injury. This is why most athletes begin to contract the fibers of an injured muscle just as soon as the pain subsides.

How to stimulate circulation with moist heat and liniment

Frequent applications of moist heat followed by massage with a warming liniment will speed healing of an injured muscle by

stimulating circulation. Towels wrung out in hot water, fomentations made from flannel, or a hot-water bottle wrapped in a moist
towel will provide adequate heat. The rays of an infrared bulb can
be used to keep a moist towel hot for 20 minutes or longer.

A formula for homemade liniments

Oil of wintergreen, also called menthyl salicylate, is a common
ingredient of liniments. You can mix wintergreen and mineral oil
for a good massage lubricant. One-half cup of oil of wintergreen
mixed with one-half cup of camphor and soap liniment makes a
liniment similar to that sold in drug stores. Plain mustard,
turpentine, or any other irritant rubbed on the skin will stimulate
circulation.

Practitioners of Russian folk medicine make an effective pain-
reducing salve by mixing 50 grams of dry camphor and 50 grams
of dry mustard with ten grams of alcohol and the whites of six
eggs. The mixture is rubbed on the skin and then removed 15
minutes later with a warm, moist towel.

Salt, dry mustard, and kerosene are sometimes mixed together
and rubbed on the skin. Even horseradish has been mixed in an
equal amount of kerosene for use as a liniment. With a little
imagination, you can concoct all kinds of liniments. All you need
is a mixture that will produce a little harmless reddening. All
liniments are *counterirritants,* which produce *irritation on the skin
in order to relieve deep pain and soreness.* If you do make your
own liniments, be careful not to make them so strong that you
blister your skin. If you prefer, you can purchase a ready-made
liniment in any drug store.

How to bathe away muscle soreness

For simple muscle soreness caused by overwork or too much
exercise, soak in a tub of hot water (about 105 degrees Fahrenheit) that contains a little mustard or oil of wintergreen. Contract
the sore muscles repeatedly during and after the bath to pump out
accumulated waste products. Finish the bath with a cool-water
rinse and vigorous rubbing with a coarse towel.

Three Simple Treatments for Midnight Leg Cramps

Patricia C. is occasionally awakened during the night with a muscle spasm in one of her calves. "The first time I had one of those spasms," she said, "the pain was so severe that I went to the emergency room at the hospital. The doctor there said that it was a muscle spasm and gave me a shot."

Patricia told me that she was still having the muscle spasm, and that they frequently lasted an hour or two. I advised her to take a calcium supplement to guard against a mineral deficiency. Then I told her to follow these instructions when a spasm occurred:

1. Stand at arm's length from a wall, place both hands on the wall, and then lean forward while keeping both feet flat on the floor. Be sure to keep your knees locked out straight so that a stretch will be placed on the muscles on the back of your calves. Try to maintain the stretch for a minute or two. Most muscle spasms can be relieved if the muscle is stretched when the spasm first begins.

2. If the spasm is already too severe and too painful to withstand stretching, wrap the leg in a hot, moist towel and massage the muscle through the towel.

3. If nothing else helps, sit in a tub of hot water and massage the leg while extending your foot (lifting the front part of your foot toward your shin) to stretch the calf muscles.

"I still have the spasm occasionally," Patricia reported later, "but I can usually stop it very quickly with one of the treatments you recommended."

Note: At the first sign of a muscle spasm in the lower leg, do something about it. Once the spasm becomes severe, it cuts off the flow of blood to the muscle and causes an even more severe spasm

If you have nightly leg cramps caused by hardened arteries, be sure to follow the instructions outlined in Chapter 1.

How to Care for Shin Splints and Arch Strains

With all the increased emphasis on walking and jogging these days, there has been an increase in the number of shin splints and arch strains. Without proper care, these two disorders can cause pain and disability that may last for many months.

How to wrap a shin splint

When a shin splint occurs, a muscle or membrane pulls away from the shin bone, so that pain occurs on the front of the leg during walking. Rest and the application of heat will speed recovery. Athletes very often apply a warming liniment or analgesic balm over the skin and then wrap the leg with an elastic bandage. A piece of foam rubber about six inches long and two inches wide placed over the shin and held in place by a bandage will provide a firm, cushioned support that will allow contraction of the muscles without obstructing the circulation of blood.

Temporary support for a painful arch

When a normal arch has been strained, a little support with a cork or rubber arch support may be enough to relieve the pain of weight bearing. Wrapping the ankle and the arch with a two-inch elastic bandage may offer adequate support until the strained ligaments heal. A contrast foot bath, such as that described in Chapter 4, will speed healing.

Summary

1. In any kind of muscle or joint injury, it's best to apply cold during the first 12 to 24 hours and wait at least 36 hours before applying heat.
2. A sprained ankle should be elevated and wrapped between applications of cold.
3. Cold reduces bleeding by constricting blood vessels. Heat speeds healing by increasing the flow of blood.
4. An effective cold pack can be made by filling a plastic bag with crushed ice and then wrapping it in a moist or dry towel.
5. A hot compress can be made by wrapping moist, hot flannel in dry flannel.
6. Excessive bruising and bleeding can be controlled with an increased intake of Vitamin C.
7. Joint strains should be rested for several days, but injured muscles can be exercised as soon as the pain subsides.
8. Massaging an injured muscle with a cylinder of ice will permit

early exercise as well as cut down on bleeding deep within the muscles.

9. Liniments and analgesic balms applied over an injured muscle prior to wrapping with an elastic bandage will speed recovery and reduce disability.

10. Muscle spasms in the lower leg can very often be relieved by stretching the muscle or by massaging it with a hot, moist towel.

6

How to Relieve Neck, Arm, and Shoulder Pain with Drugless Methods of Naturomatic Healing

Many things can cause pain in the neck, the shoulder, and the arm, but when all three body parts are involved at the same time it usually has a special meaning. You probably can decide for yourself what is causing your pain after reading this chapter, and then use the appropriate natural remedy.

How to Recognize and Relieve a Pinched Neck Nerve

When Lucas C. came into my office complaining of neck and shoulder pain that was accompanied by numbness in his thumb and forefinger, I had a good idea of what was wrong before I started examining him. Any time pain or numbness travels from the neck to one hand and involves only two or three fingers, it's a safe bet that a nerve in the neck is being pinched or irritated. X-ray examination of Lucas' neck revealed that a degenerated disc had allowed two of his vertebrae to come too close together. As a result, a bony spur had formed and was pressing against a nerve.

I recommended that Lucas C. try cervical traction, which is a simple neck-stretching treatment that may be used safely at home.

Although the pain disappeared while the traction was being applied, it took several weeks of regular use of the traction before both the pain and the numbness were completely gone. "I used the traction twice each day for six weeks," he reported, "and now I feel as good as new."

Properly applied neck traction is completely harmless. So don't hesitate to use it if you have arm pain or numbness that you suspect is being caused by a pinched nerve.

How to use neck traction

You can purchase a cervical traction apparatus in any surgical supply store and in many drug stores. It usually consists of an overhead pulley and a harness that fits around the head and under the chin. A weight is attached to the loose end of a cord that runs from the harness and over the pulley. A steady pull on the neck stretches tight neck muscles and relieves nerve pressure by pulling the bones of the neck apart just a little.

Neck traction may be applied in a sitting position or in a lying-down position, whichever is most convenient for you. If you do a lot of traveling, or if you want to use the traction in an office, you can get a special pulley arrangement that can be hooked over a door for a quick sitting stretch. I know a number of office workers who occasionally use traction "on the job" to relieve neck and arm pain caused by arthritis. (See Figure 4.)

How to make a homemade head harness for neck traction

Lucas C. made his own head harness after seeing one in my office. He purchased a three-inch wide strip of soft leather about three feet long and sewed the two ends together to make a circular band. He looped one side of the band under his chin and the other side under the back of his head and then connected each side with a narrow strip placed just below each ear. Once you get the general idea, you can add your own refinements in constructing a head harness. Sash cord or clothesline attached to the loops that extend above the head will make a good traction cord.

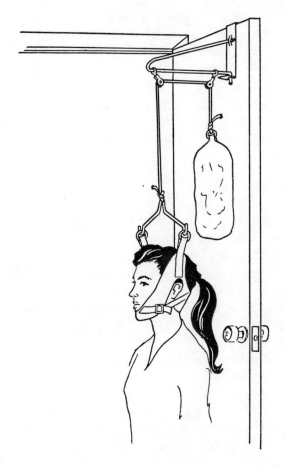

Drawing by Bibiana Neal

Figure 4. Details of a homemade head harness.

Selecting the right amount of weight

When you first begin to use neck traction, use only about five pounds for fifteen minutes. If no ill effects occur, use ten pounds for about fifteen minutes. After you have been using traction for several days, you may begin to use a heavier weight for a shorter period of time. For example, you may use fifteen pounds for ten minutes or less, or you may use seven pounds for an hour or longer. Be guided by the way you feel. Select the amount of weight that feels best to you and then use it as often or as long as necessary to provide relief from pain. Some patients report relief with as much as 25 pounds for only a few minutes at a time.

Whenever you begin to experience discomfort during traction, either reduce the amount of weight you use or decrease the time. If the weight is too heavy or the time too long, the neck muscles will tense up in resistance to the traction. It's important that the muscles be as relaxed as possible for maximum benefit in spinal stretching.

Barbell plates make convenient weights to use in traction. Or you may simply fill a couple of bags with sand. Lucas C. put brick fragments in a plastic bucket.

How to Recognize and Relieve Neck-Muscle Arm Pain

Arthur F. complained of numbness and tingling that seemed to affect his entire right arm. "It comes and goes, Doctor," he explained. "Sometimes during the night, or when I'm just standing around, my arm gets numb. The numbness goes away when I put my arms over my head."

I asked Arthur F. to stand erect with his arms at his sides and turn his head as far to the left as he could. After several seconds in this position, he began to complain of numbness in his right arm. I felt the pulse in his right wrist and found that it was barely detectable. When he turned his head back to the right and lifted his arm a little, the numbness disappeared and the pulse came back good and strong. "You either have an extra rib in your neck," I told him, "or there's a muscle pressing on a blood vessel."

X-ray examination did not reveal a neck rib, so it was apparent that a neck muscle was at fault (scalenus anticus syndrome).

I advised Arthur F. to maintain good posture, to avoid carrying heavy weights, and to occasionally stand in a doorway and press against the top door jamb with both hands. Every time he began to feel the numbness in his arm, he was to hold his arm over his head for several seconds or rest both hands on his hips. His trouble finally disappeared when improved posture and better muscle tone lifted up his sagging shoulder girdle.

How to Relieve Elbow-Pressure Neuritis

Leonard E. complained of occasional numbness in his little finger on each hand. X-ray examination did not reveal any abnormality in his neck, so I asked him if he ever sat with pressure on his elbows. "I sure do," he replied. "I work in an office, and my elbows are either on top of my desk or on my chair arms."

Leonard's little-finger numbness was being caused by constant pressure against the ulnar nerve on the inside of each elbow. Many people who sleep on their back with their elbows on the mattress and their hands on their abdomen develop such numbness during the night. It's also a common complaint among persons confined to wheel chairs or rocking chairs.

All you have to do to relieve elbow-pressure neuritis is to remove the pressure on your elbows. Persons who cannot change their sleeping posture may have to place foam rubber cushions under both elbows to relieve the pressure.

Don't ignore the simple remedies for such complaints as elbow-pressure neuritis. I've seen patients spend hundreds of dollars seeking a cause and a cure for numbness in their little fingers, only to discover years later that all they needed was a cushion under their elbows.

How to Relieve the Spasm of a Locked Neck

Few people escape an occasional "neck crick." When your neck does stiffen, there's plenty that you can do to relieve your discomfort. Most of the time, a neck crick is caused by a muscle spasm, which may result from nervous tension, an awkward movement, or a muscle strain. Occasionally, a bone in the neck will be pulled out of alignment by an awkward movement. The majority of cricks seem to occur after an awkward sleeping posture strains a joint or pulls a muscle during a deep sleep.

How moist heat application
helped Jasper on a camping trip

Jasper J. went on a camping trip and woke up the very first morning with a stiff neck. It got so bad on the second day that he drove to a telephone and called my office for advice. "The pain is on the right side of my neck where my neck and shoulder come together," he said, "and it feels as if someone is jabbing me with a knife when I move my head." When I learned that there was no pain or numbness in his arm and that he could turn his head freely to the left, I told him that he probably had a simple muscle spasm that would respond to moist heat applications.

Jasper decided to continue with his camping trip. When he returned a week later, he dropped by to tell me that the spasm lasted only four days. "I was ready to check into a hospital," he said, "until I started using that moist heat. It certainly relieved my pain in a hurry."

Simple moist heat in the form of fomentation (see Chapter 7) is more effective than pills and potions in relieving a stiff neck caused by muscle spasm. There is, however, a simple manipulation that you can use to make sure that a neck bone isn't locked.

How to test for muscle spasm

There is a simple way to tell if your neck pain is being caused by muscle spasm. If the pain is on one side of the neck and the upper back, and the pain is increased by turning the head *toward* the painful side, you know that muscles are locking the joints of your neck. A vertebra will occasionally get out of place and lock the neck, but most of the time it is the muscle that is at fault.

How to manipulate your own neck

At the first sign of a neck crick, place one hand on each side of your neck and rotate your neck *away* from the painful side. Just turn your head as far as you can and then use your hands to force a little additional rotation of your neck bones. This will unlock the joints of your neck without aggravating the muscle spasm.

Note: It's important that you use your hands to rotate your *neck* and *not* your head.

How to relax tight neck muscles
with moist heat

Wring out a towel in a basin of hot faucet water and drape it over the back of your neck. When the towel cools off, wring it out for another application. Do this at least half a dozen times. You can prolong the heat of each application by wrapping the towel in flannel or by using flannel (or a piece of part-woolen blanket) instead of towels. Running a heavy stream of hot water over your neck during a shower provides a good combination of heat and massage.

Note: During cool weather, turn up your collar or keep your neck covered with a scarf so that the spastic muscles won't be exposed to cold wind. A chill can further inflame and aggravate a muscle spasm, particularly in the neck.

How to support
your neck with a pillow

If you have trouble getting your neck into a comfortable position during the night, fluff up the bottom edge of your pillow so that it will support the back of your neck. You may have to experiment a little in order to find a position that will relieve the pain.

With proper care, the muscle spasm that causes a crick should not last longer than three or four days. It's important that you begin using simple, natural remedies just as soon as you notice the first signs of a stiff neck. Otherwise, a chronic stiff neck may result from muscle inflammation caused by unrelieved muscle spasm.

Bursitis Can Occur in Almost Any Joint

If you've never had bursitis, count your blessings. Chances are, however, that you'll eventually experience the agony of bursitis. It's most common in the shoulder, but it occurs quite often in the hip, knee, and elbow.

Knee bursitis

Generally speaking, bursitis is an inflammation of the lubricating sac that surrounds a joint. When it occurs as a swelling on the front of the knee, it is sometimes called *housemaid's knee*. This type of bursitis is commonly seen in women who get down on their hands and knees to scrub or wax floors. If you must crawl around on your knees for some reason, be sure to protect your knees with thick padding.

Bursitis on the back of the knee is called *Baker's cyst*. When you begin to feel a little tenderness or swelling behind your knee, don't sit with your legs crossed—and don't do any toe-touching exercises.

Elbow bursitis

Bursitis on the back of the elbow is called *olecranon bursitis;* when it's chronic and there is a "bump" on the tip of the elbow, it's called *miner's elbow*. Repeated injury or bumping of the elbow is usually responsible for both these conditions.

Radiohumeral bursitis

Bursitis that occurs on the outside of the elbow is called radiohumeral bursitis. Since this form of bursitis is so common, it will be discussed in more detail under the heading of "tennis elbow."

Hip bursitis

Strain or injury of the hip sometimes results in *trochanteric bursitis*. One of the worst cases of hip bursitis I have ever seen occurred in a 35-year-old sedentary man who had spent a couple of hours jumping on a trampoline. Once the bursa of a hip becomes inflamed, recovery is slow and painful. So be careful not to subject your hips to prolonged, unaccustomed strain.

Tailbone bursitis

Even the lowly tailbone can play host to bursitis, which may be called *coccygodynia*. This painful and embarrassing condition is often caused by sitting in a slumped posture on a hard surface, so that there is excessive pressure on the tailbone. In acute cases, it may be necessary to sit on a rubber ring or a doughnut-shaped cushion to relieve pressure on the bottom of the spine. A wide strap around the hips may protect the tailbone by not allowing the buttocks to spread apart while sitting. It's better to sit in a firm chair than in an overstuffed sofa, and it's absolutely necessary to sit bolt upright.

General measures for
relief from bursitis

Most forms of bursitis will respond to moist heat, rest, and light massage. When heat seems to cause an increase in pain, cold applications should be used. There are some special procedures that you must follow in the treatment of shoulder bursitis if you are to avoid permanent disability.

A Step-By-Step Self-Help Program for Relieving Acute
and Chronic Shoulder Bursitis and Tendonitis

Elizabeth B., a middle-aged housewife, woke up one morning complaining of an ache in her right shoulder. It wasn't very bad, but she had some difficulty getting her arm high enough to comb her hair. A few days later, the pain became quite severe. She couldn't lift her arm above shoulder level, and she found it impossible to reach around in back and zip up her dress.

When Elizabeth finally did visit her doctor, the pain was nearly gone but she still couldn't lift her arm above shoulder level. An orthopedic specialist told her that adhesions had developed in her shoulder and that they might make full recovery difficult or impossible. By following the simple measures outlined in the pages to follow, however, she eventually regained full use of her arm.

If you ever develop shoulder pain that limits the use of your arm, you may be suffering from bursitis *or* tendonitis. Both have similar symptoms and require nearly the same treatment. Tendonitis is simply an inflammation of one of the tendons that surround the shoulder joint. It usually causes pain only when you move your arm in a certain direction. With prompt and proper home care, you can relieve the pain of bursitis or tendonitis, and you can prevent the stiffness that causes months of disability.

How to relieve acute shoulder pain
with cold packs

When bursitis or tendonitis is so acute that the slightest movement causes agonizing pain, a cold pack might be more effective than heat in relieving pain. A bag of crushed ice wrapped in a *dry* towel might be used. Leave the pack on the shoulder for at least half an hour for a numbing effect. If the cold seems to help, apply the pack for about 20 minutes every hour for 24 to 48 hours.

How to support your arm with a sling

An arm sling will very often provide welcome relief from acute shoulder pain. You can make such a sling with a large towel or a piece of bed sheet, or you can buy one ready-made in any drug store. Adjust the sling so that it lifts the arm just enough to relieve tension on the shoulder joint.

During the night, a pillow may be used to support the arm in a comfortable position alongside your body.

Start using heat
when the pain subsides

Recurring or chronic shoulder pain that is not severe will usually respond to moist heat applied about 20 minutes every two hours. An infrared bulb or a simple light bulb in a reflector can be used to heat a moist towel draped over the shoulder.

Although cold is usually recommended for acute shoulder pain, you should switch to heat if you find that the pain is aggravated by cold. In either case, be careful not to use extreme temperatures. Excessive heat or excessive cold might trigger inflammation in a sensitive shoulder.

How to work the stiffness
out of your shoulder

You should rest your shoulder when it's in the throes of an acute attack of bursitis or tendonitis, but you should begin moving the shoulder as soon as possible to prevent "freezing" or permanent stiffness.

Try this exercise when the pain begins to ease: Lean forward and brace the "good arm" on a table top or chair arm. Let the "bad arm" hang down loosely. Keep the muscles of the painful shoulder relaxed while you swing the arm back and forth, from side to side, and in a circle, as if it were a loosely hanging pendulum. This will keep the bursa and the tendons moving enough to prevent the formation of adhesions.

As the pain in the shoulder subsides, and you begin to recover the use of your arm, start putting your arm over your head. Reach as high as you can several times each day. If you aren't able to lift your arm by muscle action, there's a special pulley arrangement that you can use to *pull* your arm overhead.

How to use the
shoulder-pulley exercise

Attach a pulley to the top of a doorway. Run a long piece of sash cord or rubber-covered clothes line over the pulley. Place a chair in the doorway and sit down. Loop one end of the line around the wrist of the "bad arm" and then reach up and grip the line on the opposite side with the "good arm." Pull down with the "good arm" so that the arm on the painful side is hoisted over your head as far as pain will permit. Do this several times a day until you're able to get the arm all the way up without assistance. (See Figure 5.)

If you don't have time to rig up a pulley, you can work your arm over your head by walking your fingers up a wall. The important thing is to make sure that you put your arm over your head at least once daily. You should stop when you feel pain, however, so that you won't wedge a swollen tendon up under a ridge of bone. This wedging can sometimes be relieved by having someone press down on your shoulder while your arm is being lifted.

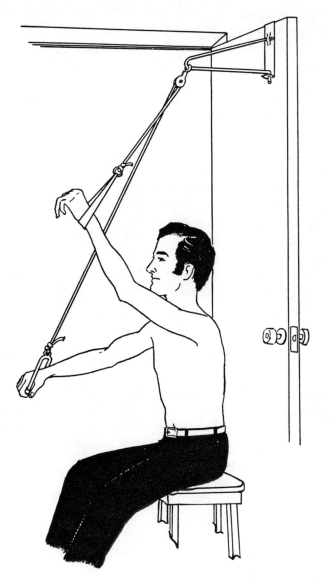

Drawing by Bibiana Neal

Figure 5. Details of a shoulder-pulley exerciser.

How to Relieve the Tendonitis
of "Tennis Elbow"

Waldo T. had a pain on the outside of his elbow that was greatly aggravated when he tried to turn a door knob, shake hands, or lift something. He could not even pick up a cup of coffee when his wrist was turned a certain way. Waldo had "tennis elbow," which is an inflammation of a bursa or, more often, a tendon attachment. "It started after I used a screw driver to assemble a book case," he said.

This painful and disabling disorder can be caused by any activity that calls for vigorous use of the forearm, as in tennis, wringing out clothes, hammering nails, and so on.

Once tennis elbow develops, it's difficult to cure. Rest is the most important part of the treatment. Care should be taken not to repeat the strain that started the trouble. As in any tendonitis, cold packs may be more effective in relieving acute pain, while moist heat is best for chronic pain. Use whichever feels best. After applying heat, put a little vegetable oil on the elbow and massage the painful area lightly with your fingertips. Waldo heated wheat germ oil and rubbed his elbow with it every day for about two weeks. After that, the pain gradually disappeared without any further treatment.

How to Make a Ganglion Disappear

When Bert J. called to say that he had a growth on the back of his wrist, he was obviously worried about having cancer or some other serious disease. What he had, however, was a ganglion cyst, which is simply a fluid-filled cyst that had developed on a wrist tendon. It was obviously not attached to bone, since it could be moved around freely under the skin. A ganglion is not dangerous, but it can be unsightly, and it can cause pain by putting pressure on tendons.

If you develop such a cyst, a blow with a book, or pressure with your fingers, may get rid of it by rupturing the sac. Just turn your hand down to tighten the skin so that the cyst will be more prominent and more vulnerable to pressure. The cyst may recur after it has been ruptured, but it's worth a try before considering surgery. Grandma always walloped a ganglion cyst with the family bible. A ganglion will sometimes disappear without treatment of any type.

Summary

1. Pain or numbness in the neck or shoulder that is accompanied by numbness in two or three fingers of one hand usually means that the neck should be stretched to relieve a pinched nerve.
2. Arm numbness that occurs when you turn your head to the opposite side may mean that a sagging shoulder girdle is pressing a blood vessel in the neck.
3. Numbness in the little finger is sometimes caused by pressure against the inside of the elbow.
4. Muscle spasm in the neck is usually aggravated by turning the head *toward* the pain, and can be relieved by applying moist heat and rotating the neck *away* from the painful side.
5. Shoulder pain that limits use of the arm is usually caused by bursitis or tendonitis.
6. Acute bursitis can usually be relieved by cold applications, but chronic bursitis responds best to moist heat.
7. It may be necessary to wear an arm sling when shoulder bursitis is acute, but you should begin moving your shoulder in all directions when the pain subsides.
8. A special overhead pulley can be used to hoist the arm overhead when the shoulder begins to stiffen from bursitis or tendonitis.
9. Elbow tendonitis can be relieved by rest, heat, and vegetable-oil massage.
10. A moveable "knot" on the back of the wrist is usually a harmless ganglion cyst that can be flattened by a blow with a book.

7

How to Get Prompt Relief from Backache, Arthritis and Leg Pain with Naturomatic Healing

No one escapes an occasional backache or back strain. There are many people who suffer constantly from backache and its related disorders. According to a Social Security Survey of Disabled Adults, two out of every 100 Americans are *disabled* by back trouble.

Arthritis is another common cause of pain and disability, and it's a common cause of backache. Just about *everyone* develops some of the symptoms of arthritis after middle age. One out of every 11 Americans has arthritis that is severe enough to require medical care, and it is variously estimated that at least 50 million Americans now suffer from arthritis.

If you don't already suffer from backache or arthritis, the chances are that you will eventually. And when you do, this chapter will prove to be very helpful in relieving pain and disability.

How to Relieve Backache and Lumbago with Applications of Heat

Just about every type of backache responds to heat. There are several ways to apply heat to the back, and all provide soothing,

114

effective relief from aches and pains. After you've finished reading this chapter, try all the various heat treatments and then select those you like best.

How to use fomentations effectively

Simple moist heat is the most effective form of heat for relieving backache. Fomentations, which are made by wrapping hot, moist towels in dry flannel, offer the best method of applying moist heat. Sections of a part-woolen blanket may be used instead of towels. Flannel, or material that is 50 percent wool and 50 percent cotton, will hold heat and moisture.

Whatever type of material you use, follow this procedure: Place a large piece of dry flannel over the back. Fold a large towel or some other material to a size that's at least twelve inches square. Then roll up the material and wring it out in hot water. Unroll the steaming towel on top of the flannel-covered back, and then fold the loose edges of the flannel over the towel to seal in the heat. That's all there is to it. With a simple fomentation, you and other members of your family can get natural, drugless relief from backache without leaving your bedroom.

Note: A fomentation cools rather rapidly and must be changed frequently—at least three applications. Each time the fomentation is changed, the skin should be dried and another piece of dry flannel placed over the back. A hot application placed in direct contact with wet skin can easily result in a burn.

How to prolong the heat
of a fomentation

After a fomentation has been applied to the back, heat can be conserved and the treatment prolonged by covering both the back and the fomentation with a sheet of rubber or plastic to seal out circulating air. A heating pad laid over an insulated fomentation will keep the moist towels hot for one continuous application. The rays of an infrared lamp or bulb can also be used to keep a fomentation hot.

George C., who works in a factory that manufactures plastic goods, finishes each day with an agonizing backache that can be completely relieved with flannel fomentations. "Until you told me how to use those hot packs," he said, "my back used to hurt until I went to bed each night. But not anymore. That new treatment gives me such relief that I've started doing a little fishing after working hours."

Warning: Do not attempt to maintain a self-heating fomentation for longer than half an hour. Prolonged exposure to heat may result in a loss of skin sensitivity that could lead to a burn. This is one reason why so many people wake up with a blister after sleeping with an electric heating pad.

How to Make a Flaxseed Poultice for Sealed-In Moist Heat

A flaxseed poultice will retain heat and moisture long enough for an effective back treatment.

Boil one cup of flaxseed in one and one-half cups of water until it has a doughy consistency. Then remove the pot from the stove, add one-half teaspoon of soda bicarbonate, and beat thoroughly to mix it with air. Spread the mixture about one inch thick between two pieces of warm muslin that are large enough to cover the painful portion of your back. Fold the edges over to prevent leakage. If you want to move about while the poultice is being applied, you can strap it to your back with a wide strip of cloth.

This poultice will stay warm for 30 to 45 minutes. One application for this period a couple of times a day should be adequate for desired pain relief.

When the poultice is removed, wash your back with warm soap and water and dry with a coarse towel. Have someone rub your back with vegetable oil and then cover it with warm flannel.

Note: Oiling the skin lightly *before* applying a poultice or plaster will help protect the skin from blistering or chapping.

Be sure to fill the empty flaxseed pot with water so that it won't be difficult to clean later.

The Mustard-Plaster Technique for Pain-Relieving Effects

A mustard plaster can be applied over the back with the same technique used to apply a flaxseed poultice.

To make a mustard plaster for an adult, mix one part mustard with four to six parts of flour in just enough *warm* water to make a smooth paste. (For a child, use one part mustard to 12 parts flour. Spread the paste about a quarter of an inch thick between two sheets of warm muslin.

The moisture in the plaster causes the mustard to release an irritating oil that generates heat by reddening the skin. You must be careful, however, not to blister the skin. Lift the plaster every five minutes and examine the skin for redness. Remove the plaster as soon as a definite pinkness appears—usually after five to 20 minutes.

When the plaster is removed, be sure to wash and dry the skin, and then oil it to prevent chapping.

Note: Remember that if mustard is exposed to a temperature above 140 degrees Fahrenheit, it won't release the oil that is responsible for the heating effect. If you prepare your mustard plasters over a stove in order to keep them warm, make sure that you don't allow them to get too hot.

How to Use a Bed Board to Support a Painful Back

"I've been sleeping on a board for three weeks," said Lamar B., a paper mill worker, "and my back hurts more now than it did when I started." And no wonder. He had placed the board on *top* of the mattress rather than under the mattress.

When a doctor recommends a bed board, he means for it to be placed between the mattress and the springs. A sheet of plywood that is at least one-half inch thick will do. Cut the board so that it will be a little smaller than the mattress and then round the corners of the board. This will prevent injury caused by sharp or projecting corners.

I advised Lamar to put the board *under* his mattress. Two days later, he called to say that his back trouble was much improved. "I rest and sleep better," he said. "My back no longer bothers me during the night, and I'm getting along better during the day. My wife likes the board, too, and she now wants to sleep in *my* bed."

If you have any type of back trouble, or if your back seems to be sore and stiff when you get out of bed in the morning, use a bed board. It might be the answer to your aching back problem.

A good mattress is important

A simple cotton or felt mattress may be better than a thick, expensive inner-spring mattress. A mattress that's too hard, however, can be very uncomfortable. Make sure that there is just enough "give" in the mattress to conform to the contours of your body without sagging in the middle.

Support your knees with a pillow

There are many types of back trouble that can be aggravated by lying on your back with your legs flat on the mattress. Whenever you experience such discomfort in spite of having a good mattress, place a thick pillow under both knees so that you can rest with your knees bent. This will relieve the tension in certain hip muscles that attach to the bones of the lower spine, thus allowing the spine to relax. .

How to Stretch Your Lower Back to Relieve Sciatic Neuritis

Crawford J. complained of leg ache and numbness that radiated down the outside of his right calf into the top of his foot and his big toe. "I hurt my back several years ago," he said, "but my back isn't bothering me now—just my leg." Examination revealed that an old ruptured disc was pressing against a nerve that traveled from his back to his foot. "I'd be willing to try anything to avoid surgery or to keep from going to the hospital," Crawford J. said with desperation. I recommended spinal traction that could be used at home. The leg pain disappeared after only two weeks of using the traction.

When pain or numbness seems to radiate from your back into your thigh or leg, it may mean that a spinal nerve is being pinched or irritated by an arthritic spur or a ruptured disc. In either case, stretching your lower spine may relieve the pain for you just as it did for Crawford—by pulling the vertebrae apart far enough to relieve pressure on the swollen nerve.

Moist heat applied to the lower back before using the traction will relieve spasm and soreness for more effective stretching. It may be necessary to combine many of the treatment methods recommended in this chapter for permanent relief from pain.

How to rig low-back traction with a pelvic harness

Most surgical supply stores can provide you with a special pelvic harness that can be used to stretch your lower spine. A weight is attached to the end of a cord that runs from the harness and over a pulley that is fastened to the foot of the bed. You can purchase a pulley apparatus that can be clamped to the mattress or hooked over a foot board—or you can construct your own pulley arrangement. (See Figure 6.)

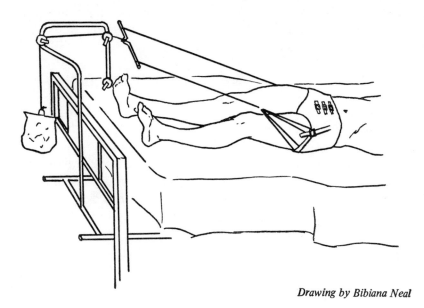

Drawing by Bibiana Neal

Figure 6. Details for a pelvic harness.

Place a couple of bricks under the foot of the bed so that it will be elevated several inches. Then adjust the pulley apparatus so that the traction cord pulls up at an angle of 30 degrees or so. A pillow placed under both knees will flex the hips slightly so that the traction will be more effective.

Selecting the right amount of weight

Begin your traction by using about 15 pounds for half an hour. If no ill effects result, gradually work up to 25 pounds or more. Use the traction at least twice a day. Whenever time and comfort permit, you may use the traction for any length of time you desire. Pelvic traction is completely safe, but it shouldn't be used when a pull on an injured spinal joint causes pain.

Barbell plates are commonly used for weight in pelvic traction, but a sandbag or a water bag will be less likely to damage the bed or the floor.

You won't have any trouble getting into traction by yourself if you'll make the traction cord long enough to let the weight rest on the floor when the traction is not being used. Just scoot down to the foot of the bed to slip on the harness and then move back toward the head of the bed to lift the weight from the floor.

How to Relieve Back and Leg Pain with Sofa Traction

If you don't have a harness and a pulley for stretching out back and leg pain, use this sofa technique: Lie down on the floor and drape your legs over the arm of a sofa. Scoot up close to the sofa so that your thighs are nearly vertical. For best results, the support of the sofa should be just high enough to lift your hips an inch or two off the floor. When necessary, a pillow placed over the arm of a sofa will provide a little additional lift.

Sofa traction relieves pressure on joints and nerves by placing a slight pull on the lower back and by reversing the weight-bearing posture of the spine. Lying on your side and rolling up into a ball by pulling your knees to your chest has a similar effect in relieving leg pain caused by nerve pressure.

Special Support for a Painful Back

When a low-back strain is so severe that movement is difficult or painful, a special support may help you. Pain near the center of the lower back is usually in the lumbosacral joints and calls for a *lumbosacral corset.*

If you have recurring back trouble that's caused by an unstable spine or a "slipped disc," you might occasionally benefit from temporary support. For example, a patient of mine, Lee B., carries his corset with him when he travels. When his back "goes out," he slips the corset on and wears it until the spasm subsides. Tim J. cannot afford to miss any time at work because of a bad back, so he is forced to wear a corset occasionally in order to stay on the job.

A lumbosacral corset can be purchased in surgical supply stores and in some drug stores. Many large department stores sell a lady's corset that is especially designed to support a bad back.

When back pain is low on one side of the pelvis (in the "hip" area) and causes a limp on the painful side, you need a *sacroiliac belt* for a sacroiliac strain.

Note: It's not a good idea to wear a corset or a back support after the pain and spasm subside. Unnecessary or prolonged use of a back support may weaken muscles and increase chances of injury.

How to Use Heat and Massage to Chase Out Fibromyositis and Muscular Inflammation

Soreness around the upper back is often caused by postural strain, nervous tension, exposure to chilling wind, and other factors that inflame the muscles. When soreness is chronic, it's often called myositis, fibrositis, or fibromyositis.

If you suffer from tension and postural strain, be sure to study the tension-relief techniques described in Chapter 3 and the posture rules outlined in Chapter 4. In the meantime, pain and spasm in inflamed muscles can be relieved with moist heat and massage. Vitamin E taken orally seems to help. Some researchers claim good results from rubbing Vitamin E-rich wheat germ oil into the skin over painful muscles.

How to combine heat, massage, and exercise for pain relief

Apply hot fomentations to the sore muscles for about half an hour. Then massage the muscles with cocoa butter, vegetable oil, or mineral oil. A little oil of wintergreen mixed with the lubricant will leave the skin warm and pink. Use the heat and massage at least once daily. After each massage, shrug your shoulders up and down and then wave your arms back and forth at shoulder level, so that muscular contraction will pump out waste products that have been loosened by the massage. Remember that progress in the treatment of chronic fibromyositis is slow, so don't give up if you don't notice much improvement after the first few days.

A television personality who endured great tension day after day reported that the simple program I have just outlined relieved soreness and stiffness that had persisted for years. "I used the moist heat, the massage, and the muscle contraction every night for a month," she said. "My muscles no longer ache and burn, but I still use the treatment a couple of times a week just to keep my muscles healthy." If you don't get plenty of regular exercise, you should heat, massage, and contract your muscles at least twice a week.

How to Relieve the Pain and Stiffness
of Arthritis and Rheumatism

Pain caused by spinal arthritis can be relieved by any of the measures already described for the relief of backache. Moist heat applications are effective in the treatment of arthritis anywhere in the body. In the arms and legs, however, where small, bony surfaces are hard to heat evenly, a paraffin bath may be more effective. You can use ordinary household paraffin, which can be purchased in any grocery store.

The Technique of Using a Paraffin Bath

Melt four pounds of paraffin and one-half pint of mineral oil in the top of an ordinary double boiler. For larger amounts, mix four parts paraffin to one part mineral oil. If you have a bath or candy thermometer, adjust the temperature of the melted paraffin to 125 to 130 degrees. If you don't have a thermometer, let the paraffin cool until a film forms on the surface before applying it to your body. You can test the temperature by inserting a stick of paraffin into the melted paraffin. If the stick melts, the paraffin is too hot.

How to put a paraffin glove
on a hand or a foot

When you have arthritis in a hand or a foot, a paraffin dip will provide quick and effective relief from soreness and stiffness. The hand, for example, can be dipped in the paraffin several times to form a thick, insulating glove that literally seals in heat and moisture. After one quick dip has been made and the hand is covered with a protective coat of paraffin, each successive dip can be prolonged for a greater heating effect. Pause just long enough between dips for each new coat of paraffin to harden. Keep dipping until the paraffin is at least one-quarter of an inch thick.

When the last dip is made, immersion for several minutes will build up heat in the deeper layers of paraffin for a long-lasting heating effect. The heat can be conserved by wrapping the paraffin-coated hand in oil cloth or a dry towel. Be sure to keep your fingers still so that you won't crack the cooling paraffin.

The more oil you add to the paraffin, the lower its melting point will be. Pure paraffin has a much higher melting point and is therefore much hotter. Persons who can tolerate higher temperatures report good results with pure paraffin.

A professional golfer who has arthritis in both hands dips his hands in paraffin before every tournament. "I don't believe that I could make it without that hot wax," he said. "The ability to use my hands means money in the bank and bread on the table." If you must use your hands in sports, typing, sewing, playing a musical instrument, or in some other activity requiring use of your fingers, you may find the paraffin bath especially helpful—even job-saving.

Special note! Recent investigations have revealed that wearing a tight pair of stretch gloves while sleeping will eliminate the painful morning stiffness in arthritic hands.

How to paint your joints
with paraffin

Joints that cannot be dipped in paraffin, such as the knee, elbow, and spinal joints, can be *painted* with paraffin. A plain two-inch paint brush will do. Just keep painting until the painful joints are coated with at least a quarter-inch of paraffin. The paraffin-coated joints may then be wrapped in plastic or some other material to conserve heat. A rain coat or a sheet of flannel can be laid over the back. (See Figure 7.)

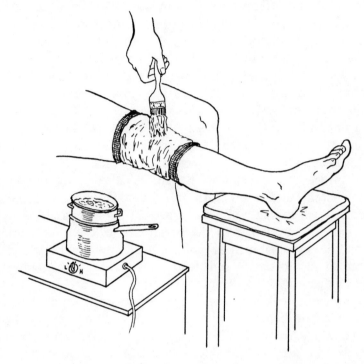

Drawing by Bibiana Neal

Figure 7. Technique of painting limbs with paraffin.

When the paraffin no longer feels warm—after 30 minutes or longer—it may be peeled from the skin and saved for use over and over again. You can clean dirty paraffin by heating it in water and then pouring off the water.

Warning: Paraffin is very flammable, so be careful not to spill any over an open flame or a heating unit. This is one of the reasons for using a double boiler—so that paraffin can be heated indirectly.

Oil or shave hairy areas before applying paraffin so that you won't pull out the hair when you peel off the paraffin. If you have trouble getting the first coat of paraffin to stick to smooth or oily skin, you can wrap the joint with a layer of gauze before painting on the first coat. The gauze will serve as an anchor sheet.

How to Heat All of Your Muscles and Joints with a Cabinet Bath

Grover L. was a retired carpenter who complained of aches and pains all over his body. In addition to generalized arthritis, he seemed to be suffering from inflammation of nerves and muscles, which doctors often call neuritis or myositis—or just plain rheumatism. "Every muscle and joint in my body aches," he said with suffering resignation. Rather than attempt to apply heat to every portion of his body separately, I suggested that he build himself a light-bulb baker so that he could heat his entire body with an even temperature for at least half an hour at a time.

Several months later, Grover L. called to say that he had built the baker and that he was using it regularly. "It works fine," he said. "Thirty minutes in the baker each morning relieves my stiffness enough to get me through the day with very little pain. I've even built a few extra bakers and sold them to friends."

How to make your own "pain baker"

You can make a baker with little or no trouble. Just build a half-circle or half-octagon frame that will reach from your neck to your feet. Line it with reflecting aluminum or tin foil and put in a couple rows of evenly-spaced light bulbs. The reflector should be at least 18 inches away from your body on all sides when you are lying under the baker. You can control the heat by using certain size light bulbs or by lighting a certain number of bulbs.

It might be a good idea to leave each end of the baker open to allow the circulation of air so that sweating won't be excessive. A cold pack placed over your forehead will help prevent overheating.

Lie relaxed under the baker for about half an hour once or twice a day. Follow each baking with a warm shower that's gradually turned down to a cool temperature—or at least rub your skin with a cool, moist wash cloth.

How to Keep Arthritis from Stiffening Your Joints

During acute attacks of arthritis, when movement is painful and the joints are swollen and inflamed, rest and cold applications may be best for relief from pain. But when arthritis becomes chronic, the affected joints should be put through a full range of movement several times a day—preferably after applying heat or following a hot bath. Remember this rule: *An arthritic joint should be used just enough to prevent stiffness and the formation of adhesions but not so much that a painful reaction occurs.*

Don't participate in strenuous, unaccustomed activities. Begin any new activity lightly and progressively so that you can evaluate the effects of the activity from day to day. If you find, for example, that your joints are sore and stiff the day after exercising, you'll know that you did too much.

How Lillian coped with her chronic arthritis

Lillian J. first began to notice a little joint stiffness after her fortieth birthday. "I would feel stiff when I first got up in the morning," she said. "And if I sat for very long, I would be really stiff for awhile. Exercise makes me feel better, but if I do too much I'm so sore and stiff the next day that I can hardly move."

Lillian had chronic arthritis. Once she learned how to limit her activities and then use simple home treatment to ease the pain during acute attacks, she got along fine. "I don't get nearly as sore and stiff as I once did," she said happily. "In fact, I'm hardly even aware that I have arthritis. The treatment you recommended really does the trick."

Home-treatment methods offer the best possible approach to the care of arthritis. If you'll study this chapter carefully and then put into practice what you learn, chances are you won't be crippled with stiff joints.

How to combine heat and liniment for special benefits

When an arthritic joint flares up, apply moist heat and then rub the joint with oil of wintergreen and alcohol that has been mixed to a suitable strength. Wrapping the joint in flannel will maintain the warmth generated by the liniment.

The muscles surrounding a painful arthritic joint may be massaged, and it may be all right to use light fingertip massage over the joint, but you should never use a vibrator over a joint that is throbbing with pain.

How to use an infrared bulb

Heat from the rays of an infrared bulb (which can be clamped to the back of a chair) is a convenient and effective way to apply heat to an arthritic joint before and after exercise. You can purchase one of these bulbs in any drug store.

How to relieve deformity with a
firm mattress and good posture

If you have rheumatoid arthritis, be careful not to let the affected joints stiffen in a slumped or bent position. A bed patient, for example, who lies with his spine sagging and his knees bent may find that his posture is permanently distorted when he leaves the bed.

Make sure that your mattress does not sag. Lie straight and flat; sit and stand straight. *If you have knee or hip arthritis, don't sleep with a pillow under your knees to relieve an aching back.* A head pillow that's too high may also be harmful for an arthritic spine.

How to loosen a stiff spine

Traction on the neck and the lower back, as described in Chapter 6 and in this chapter, will sometimes relieve spinal stiffness. The upper back manipulation described in Chapter 3 is very effective for loosening the vertebrae between the shoulder blades. The neck manipulation described in Chapter 6 will help restore a normal range of movement in the joints of the neck.

There is a special loosening movement that you can use on your lower spine. Lie on your back with your feet off the floor and your knees and hips flexed at right angles to each other. Hold your legs together in this position and drop them first to one side and then to the other by twisting at your waist. Keep your upper back flat on the floor so that the lower spine will be forced to rotate. Place your hands palms-down on the floor on each side for counterbalance. (See Figure 8.)

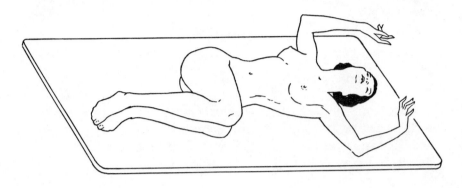

Drawing by Bibiana Neal

Figure 8. Technique for loosening the lower spine.

You can learn more about the care of backache in my book *Backache: Home Treatment and Prevention* (Parker Publishing Company, West Nyack, New York 10994).

How Good Nutrition Helps Arthritis and Backache

No matter what type of arthritis you have, good nutrition should be part of the treatment. A variety of fresh, *natural* foods supplies essential vitamins and minerals. Plenty of fresh fruits and vegetables will alkalize the blood as well as supply nourishment. Vitamin C helps rebuild damaged joint cartilage. Vitamin C and manganese has been recommended for strengthening a "bad disc." Vitamin B helps the function of the adrenal glands, which control joint inflammation. Vitamin E may help prevent the formation of adhesions. And Vitamin D, which functions with calcium and phosphorus, helps rebuild bone. Practically every vitamin and mineral you can name plays a part in building the total body health you need to combat arthritis. So it's important that you have a good, nutritious diet.

Occasionally supplement your diet with brewer's yeast, desiccated liver, wheat germ oil, natural Vitamin C, cod liver oil, and other basic natural food supplements. *Cut out the use of white sugar and other refined foods,* particularly those containing chemical additives. Expose your aching joints to the sun's rays for Vitamin D and healing heat.

Summary

1. Fomentations made with flannel that has been wrung out in hot water provide effective moist heat for backache and arthritis.
2. A flaxseed poultice over the back seals in heat and moisture for a good half-hour heat treatment.
3. A mustard plaster applied to the back for several minutes will relieve pain through a process called counterirritation.
4. A half-inch-thick sheet of plywood placed between the mattress and the springs will relieve backache by supporting a sagging spine.
5. Back pain that radiates into the leg can very often be relieved by stretching the lower spine with a special harness.
6. Chronic muscle soreness can be relieved with a combination of heat, massage, and muscle contraction.
7. Melted paraffin can be painted over an arthritic joint, and it can be used as a "dip" for the hands and the feet.
8. If you ache all over, you can benefit from a home-made baker made from a frame lined with tin foil and light bulbs.
9. An arthritic joint should be put through a full range of movement each day so that it won't become permanently stiff.
10. Vitamin C, Vitamin D, calcium, and other vitamins and minerals supplied by *natural* foods are important in the treatment of chronic muscle and joint pains.

8

Tested Naturomatic Healing
Methods for Headache,
Constipation and Hemorrhoids

Headache, "irregularity," and hemorrhoids are such common afflictions that they are frequently depicted in graphic TV commercials and printed advertisements promoting the use of patent medicines. All of these ailments, however, can be relieved with simple home remedies that employ drugless methods. With *natural* remedies you can get immediate, soothing relief without resorting to medication that might have side effects or result in an allergic reaction. You'll learn about these remedies in this chapter—and you can use all of them at home.

A Dozen Ways to Relieve Throbbing, Nagging Headaches

There are many causes of headache. About 90 percent of all headaches are of the tension and migraine variety—and most of these are caused by simple tension. Contraction of muscles on the back of the neck tightens joints and irritates nerves. This can cause spasm of blood vessels around the head, which results in throbbing pain that beats in rhythm with the heart beat. A *migraine-type* headache is usually a throbbing headache that involves one side of the head and is accompanied by nausea or vomiting. A *tension headache,* which is less severe than a migraine, may be a steady ache that involves the whole head or only the base of the skull.

Anything you can do to relax and loosen the muscles and vertebrae of your neck will relieve most headaches by relieving pressure on nerves and blood vessels. Very little is known about the cause of migraine headache, but there is a great deal that you can do to relieve the symptoms.

James C. was a victim of daily tension headache. "I've had these headaches for about three years," he said, "and I've been to several doctors with no results." I recommended a daily self-help program that quickly proved to be effective in relieving his symptoms. James had to use the treatment daily to relieve his recurring headaches, but you may use the treatment only when necessary to relieve an occasional headache.

Naomi R. developed a headache every time her in-laws visited her home. "It starts on the back of my head and neck," she said, "and spreads up over my head. Sometimes it feels as if I'm wearing a steel ring around my head." Naomi realized that her headaches had an emotional origin, but she wasn't able to prevent them. "Each headache holds on until I go to bed at night, and it ruins my evening."

I described several home headache treatments for Naomi and told her to use the one she liked best. She reported that the moist heat and neck massage seemed to be the most effective. "I told my husband how to massage my neck," she said, "and now every time his mother visits us I make him give me a neck massage. It works like a charm!"

The next time your neck muscles tighten from a hectic day and you feel the tension creeping up the back of your head, you can use a natural headache remedy to relieve the symptoms before they have a chance to build into a full-size headache.

How to use moist heat and massage to relax tight neck muscles

Simple moist heat applied to the back of the neck is very effective in relaxing tight neck muscles. Just wring out a towel in a basin of hot water and then drape the towel over the back of your neck. Do this three or four times in succession to assure complete relaxation with a maximum blood flow.

After heat has been applied, the neck muscles should be massaged to work out accumulated waste products and flush them into the bloodstream. There's a special technique that you should use in massaging the neck, however: attention should be concentrated on the muscle attachments at the *top* of the neck. If you were massaging someone's neck, here's how you should do it: Encircle the back of the patient's neck at the base of his skull with the thumb and forefinger of your right hand. Place the palm of your left hand on the patient's forehead. Then instruct the patient to tilt his head forward and relax his neck so that your hand supports his head. Press the massaging edge of your hand firmly against the patient's neck and then knead up and down in a short circular motion. Just move the skin over the muscles so that there won't be any friction on the surface of the skin.

How to stretch the neck
to relieve tension headache

If your headache doesn't respond to heat and massage, simple neck stretching might do the trick. The cervical traction described in Chapter 6 for the relief of arm pain caused by a pinched nerve is often very effective in relaxing tight neck muscles. If you don't have a head harness and the pulley equipment you need for mechanical traction, you may use a manual technique.

Place both hands on the back of your neck near the base of your skull. Tilt your head forward and press your hands forward and upward against the back of your head. Concentrate on stretching the muscles on the back of your neck.

If you prefer, you can have some member of your family stretch your neck. Lie down across a bed and have someone grip your neck at the base of your skull. Instruct your helper to pull slowly and smoothly until your neck is stretched as far as it will go. Keep your neck muscles as relaxed as possible while the stretch is being applied. No harm will result if the stretching is smooth rather than jerky. The pull should be released and repeated a couple of times to assure complete relaxation of muscles. Stop the stretching if you experience any discomfort. Don't be alarmed if your neck clicks or pops while your neck is being stretched. The sound you hear is merely the separation of a tight joint.

How to constrict throbbing blood vessels
with coffee and ice packs

Since many headaches are caused by expansion of blood vessels around the brain, you may be able to relieve your pain with measures that *constrict* or reduce the swollen condition of the blood vessels. The caffeine in a cup of strong coffee, for example, will very often relieve a vascular headache (caused by swollen veins). If you're too nauseated to drink the coffee, you can inject it into your rectum with a syringe or an enema tip. Retain the coffee as long as you can so that your body will have time to absorb the caffeine into the circulatory system.

An ice pack wrapped in a dry towel and placed against the front of the neck or on the forehead will sometimes do the trick. Simply immersing your hands or your feet in cold water will reflexly constrict the blood vessels around your brain. A hot foot bath, combined with a cold pack around your head or neck, will draw blood from your brain for quick relief in congestive headaches.

How to correct low blood sugar headaches
with fruit sugar

Low blood sugar is a common cause of headache. Persons who miss a meal or two, for example, frequently complain of headache that disappears after eating. A snack of almost any type of food will restore the blood sugar level. It's important, however, that you eat fresh, natural foods. The wrong kind of food—the refined variety—may actually trigger a drop in blood sugar three or four hours after eating. You'll learn more about this later in the book when you read the section dealing with fatigue.

A headache that occurs after drinking alcoholic beverages is often caused by low blood sugar. A little honey stirred into a glass of fruit juice will quickly raise blood sugar and aid your body in burning the alcohol in your system. Don't attempt to use white sugar products to raise your blood sugar level in combating a headache. Your body needs *fructose,* which is a fruit sugar found in natural fruit juices.

A little salty beef broth will restore minerals and water in tissues that have been dehydrated by alcohol (alcohol unites with water in your system). The next time you wake up with a hangover headache, have some natural fruit juice for breakfast and a portion of beef broth for lunch.

How to rid yourself of allergy headaches with an "elimination diet"

Migraine or "sick" headache is sometimes caused by a food allergy. If you develop a headache after eating a certain food item, such as chocolate or milk, you know that you must eliminate that food from your diet.

One way to determine if you have a food allergy is to restrict your diet to a couple of basic food items and then add one new food each day. When a headache occurs, the last food added to your diet may be responsible for your allergy headache.

How to stop sick headache with miscellaneous remedies

Some people find that a migraine headache can be stopped in its early stages by taking an *enema* or by *wrapping a tight bandage around the head* to compress swollen, throbbing blood vessels. Once a headache develops, it may be necessary to *rest in a dark room with your head slightly elevated.* Some therapists recommend that you take *six calcium lactate tablets every two hours.*

Light pressure on the big arteries in the neck will sometimes relieve throbbing head pain. Just locate the pulse on each side of your throat and exert a little pressure with your fingertips for a few seconds at a time. *Pressure on a swollen temporal or scalp blood vessel* is often beneficial. Persons who suffer from true migraine or a histamine headache can very often see a throbbing blood vessel on the painful side of the head.

A histamine headache is similar to a migraine headache, except that it's accompanied by a running nose and a watery eye on the side of the pain. Most histamine headaches don't last very long, but it's usually necessary to *remain in an upright position to reduce pressure in the swollen, sensitive blood vessels.*

No matter what type of headache you think you have, try all the various remedies until you find something that helps. In the case of migraine, it's best to begin using headache remedies when the warning signs appear—which may be about half an hour before the headache begins. If you have recurring migraine headache that does not seem to respond to anything you do, it may comfort you to know that *the female menopause and the male climacteric will sometimes "cure" migraine* by altering the hormone balance in the body.

Hints on the care of sinus headache

A sinus headache radiates from the bony cavities in the bones around the eyes and the nose. The pain is aggravated by moving or bending forward, but may be relieved by *lying down to permit drainage of the mucus-filled sinuses.* Inhaling steam or irrigating the nose, as described in Chapter 2, will help open clogged sinuses.

Sinus trouble is often caused by an allergy, which means that you must make every effort to breathe clean, dust-free air. A hot pack or a cold pack applied over a painful sinus will very often relieve a sinus headache. When a sinus is draining, gently blow only one side of your nose at a time so that you won't force any of the mucus back into the sinus.

Watch for carbon monoxide and fever

Carbon monoxide fumes from engines and heaters are a common cause of headache. If you aren't able to relieve your headache or determine its cause, be sure to check your car muffler and the heater vents in your home.

Headache accompanied by fever is almost always caused by infection, and may require special medication. Any headache that persists in spite of all you do to help yourself should be investigated by a doctor.

How to Overcome Constipation Without Using Laxatives

Just about everyone suffers from constipation at one time or another. But don't jump to the conclusion that you're constipated just because your bowels don't move every day. Some people don't go to the toilet as often as others. There are, in fact, some people who go only once every two or three days. Regardless of how infrequently you may go to the toilet, you are not constipated unless your stool is hard and lumpy or in the shape of marbles. If you really are constipated, there are at least four important steps that you should take to get permanent relief.

Jordan A., who had taken a laxative about twice weekly for a number of years, was able to establish satisfying regularity after only a few months of following the same four-step program I've outlined for you below. "My bowels used to move only twice a week with the aid of laxatives," he said, "but now they move normally—and I no longer take laxatives." He added that he was delighted to find that he no longer suffered from headache, fatigue, and gas pains after his bowels started to function normally.

Step 1: quit using laxatives!

Constipation is very often caused by failure to make regular visits to the toilet. It's also caused by excessive use of laxatives. In fact, almost all cases of chronic constipation are the result of habitual use of commercial laxatives.

Many people fail to realize that it may take three or four days for enough waste matter to accumulate in the lower colon to trigger an "urge" after the intestinal tract has been emptied by a laxative. As a result, they grow impatient after a few days and take another laxative. The lower bowel soon becomes accustomed to emptying only when it is stimulated by a powerful irritant, resulting in the worst kind of constipation.

A mild bark laxative. If you feel that you must taper off your use of laxatives, switch for temporary relief to *cascara sagrada,* which is a mild laxative made from the bark of a certain tree. Then gradually discontinue its use.

Step 2: visit the toilet regularly

It's very important to go to the toilet at the same time each day, preferably after eating. Never ignore an urge to empty your bowels, however. When "nature calls," you should respond immediately. Give your bowels plenty of time to move. Sit with your hips flexed and your feet on a foot stool or on a ten-inch stack of books etc. This elevated posture of the feet is naturally effective in evacuating the bowels most completely.

Step 3: take an enema
when necessary

When your bowels fail to move normally after three days, you can take a deep, cleansing enema.

Mix one teaspoon of salt and two teaspoons of sodium bicarbonate in a quart of warm water. Put the solution in an enema bag and then suspend the bag on the wall about two feet above the floor. Lie down on the floor, on your left side, with your right leg bent, and insert the lubricated enema tip three or four inches into your rectum. You can control the flow of water by manipulating a clamp on the rubber tube. If you begin to feel an urge to empty your bowels before the enema is complete, clamp off the flow of water until the urge subsides. Let the water flow slowly. After the colon is filled with water, it might be a good idea to roll over on your back and press your thighs and buttocks together in order to hold the water for several minutes. This will help soften the hard, lumpy waste matter before evacuation takes place.

Olive oil for lubrication. You can make a morning enema more effective by injecting a cup of olive oil into your rectum at bedtime. The overnight action of the oil will soften and lubricate the hardened waste matter for a smooth evacuation.

A quickie toilet enema. If your bowels persist in giving you a tough time, you can take a "quickie enema" during regular toilet visits. Just use a syringe, or a disposable enema kit (available in drug stores) to inject a pint of water into your rectum. In a particularly stubborn case, you can inject a couple ounces of warm olive oil into your rectum before a scheduled bowel movement or before an enema. In some cases, it may be necessary to carefully insert a finger into your rectum to break up a large, hard mass blocking the evacuation.

Note: Attempts to force evacuation of an impacted colon by "straining at the stool" may cause hemorrhoids or result in a painful tear or fissure in the tissue around the bowel opening. Be sure to soften the waste matter in your rectum with oil or water when necessary in stubborn constipation.

Step 4: eat moisture-retaining foods

The type of food you eat is very important in providing permanent relief from constipation. In order to make sure that your stools are moist and well formed and that you won't have to continue taking enemas, you must *drink plenty of water and juices and eat a variety of fresh fruits and vegetables.* The cellulose in the indigestible portion of fruits and vegetables will provide bulk that will retain moisture so that the waste matter in your colon won't become dry and tightly packed—provided, of course, that you have regular toilet habits. If you resist or postpone an urge for very long, your colon will absorb moisture from the waste matter, making it more difficult to evacuate.

Natural fruit laxatives. Dried fruits, such as prunes, figs, raisins, and dates, aid elimination by stimulating the bowels. A light, daily late-afternoon snack of assorted dried fruits will encourage a regular morning action the next day. Any kind of fresh fruit, in large quantities, tends to have a laxative action.

Dried prunes soaked overnight in hot water containing lemon juice and honey will yield a bowel-moving infusion. Mix it to suit your taste. Drink the liquid an hour before breakfast and then eat the prunes with a little plain yogurt during breakfast. "It never fails for me," reported an 80-year-old retired railroad conductor. "When my bowels skip a day or two, I drink a small glass of that prune juice drink and I'm usually all right again for the next few months."

Go easy on bran. The bran in whole grain cereals and bread is helpful in stimulating the bowels, but it may not be a good idea to eat pure bran cereals in large quantities. Too much bran in the diet may leave a residue that will form a dry, tightly packed mass that is difficult to move.

A special non-irritating bulk diet

If you must go on a low-residue or "soft" diet because of some type of stomach or intestinal trouble, you can add non-irritating bulk to your diet with products made from *agar-agar* and *psyllium seed extract.* These indigestible products contain a gelatinous substance that will retain water without irritating a sensitive intestine. And they'll provide the bulk you need for the formation of a moist, natural stool.

Most drug stores and health food stores sell an agar powder or a psyllium muciloid that can be mixed in drinking water. Drug store commercial products are often mixed with mineral oil for intestinal lubrication. Remember, however, that the indigestible mineral oil tends to wash oil-soluble vitamins out of the intestinal tract.

Carbohydrates, Constipation, and Cancer

In addition to causing constipation, excessive use of such refined carbohydrates as white flour and white sugar can cause cancer of the colon. *In the United States, colon cancer is reported to be the second most common cause of death from cancer.*

Recent research has revealed that concentrated carbohydrate in the colon causes bacterial changes that produce cancer-causing chemicals. In addition, the absence of bulk in the carbohydrate waste allows the cancer-causing agents to remain in the colon long enough to trigger a malignant growth. You need carbohydrates in your diet, but they should come from natural foods that contain the cellulose your bowels need to function normally. Don't clog your bowels with *processed* carbohydrates that have been commercially prepared as "convenience" or time-saving "instant" foods.

It may be true that your body does not absorb toxins from

your lower bowel. But an overloaded, clogged, and distended bowel can cause headache, nausea, abdominal distension, and other symptoms of "biliousness"—not to mention the possibility of colon cancer. So it makes good sense to take good care of your bowels. You can get along without using laxatives, and avoid the disease and discomfort that results from suffering bowels.

How to Soothe the Burning, Itching Pain of Hemorrhoids

Hemorrhoids, also called "piles," are simply varicose veins; that is, veins that are swollen, stretched, and gorged with blood. Pregnancy and straining to empty the bowels are common causes of rectal varicose veins. The enlarged veins frequently bleed and itch following a bowel movement.

When hemorrhoids occur around the outside of the bowel opening, they're called *external hemorrhoids;* when they occur up inside the bowel, they're called *internal hemorrhoids.*

External hemorrhoids probably cause the most trouble, since they are more likely to be irritated during cleaning with toilet tissue.

Gilbert U. had long been aware of some burning and itching after each bowel movement, but he didn't realize that he had hemorrhoids until he began to notice blood on his toilet tissue. "I'll do anything," he said, "to avoid surgery for hemorrhoids." Fortunately, Gilbert was a patient person who could follow instructions. He was able to keep his hemorrhoids under control with simple home-treatment methods. If you have hemorrhoids, you may be able to avoid surgical intervention by following the same program that I recommended for Gilbert.

Protect hemorrhoids with a proper diet

No matter what type of hemorrhoids you have, you must avoid constipation. Straining to empty the bowels will increase the size of the hemorrhoids by gorging or "pumping" them with blood. There shouldn't be too much roughage in the diet, either. When your hemorrhoids are giving you trouble, a low-residue diet (such as that recommended for an anal fissure) supplemented with agar or psyllium seed extract will keep your stools moist and non-irritating.

How to lubricate your hemorrhoids
with olive oil

Two or three ounces of olive oil injected into your rectum with an ordinary ear syringe will provide soothing lubrication for inflamed hemorrhoids. The oil will also coat the waste matter for an easier bowel movement. One of my patients rubs wheat germ oil on his hemorrhoids, and he claims that the Vitamin E in the oil has a healing effect.

How to clean hemorrhoids
after each bowel movement

Wash the anal area with a sponge filled with cold water. Then pat the area dry with absorbent cotton and powder it with talcum or a medicated powder.

Internal hemorrhoids can be cleaned by washing out the rectum with cold water after each bowel movement. Use a syringe to inject the water and then expel the water by contracting the muscles of your bowels. It might also be a good idea to wrap a finger in moist cotton and then insert the finger just inside the anus to clean the crevices around the opening.

How to soothe hemorrhoids
with heat

External hemorrhoids often respond to a hot hip bath or to hot towels applied between the buttocks. Pads of gauze may be soaked in hot water and applied directly against the hemorrhoids.

I asked one of my patients who has a bad case of hemorrhoids what he does to relieve his discomfort. "You won't believe this, Doctor," he replied, "but I fill a bucket with boiling hot water and a little turpentine and then sit on the bucket with my buttocks spread apart. The medicated steam bathes my hemorrhoids and gives me immediate relief."

Actually, the use of turpentine and steam in the treatment of hemorrhoids is not new. One popular ointment for hemorrhoids contains turpentine along with menthol and camphor. The use of medicated steam in treating external hemorrhoids has long been a part of European folk medicine.

How to make an anal steam bath

When hemorrhoids are sensitive and inflamed, you can apply heat and medication simultaneously with soothing steam.

Follow these instructions to make a hemorrhoid steam bath:

1. Purchase a large pail or bucket that's sturdy enough to sit on.
2. Get a smooth plank that's wider than the diameter of the bucket. Cut a six-inch hole in the center of the plank.
3. Boil about two gallons of water that contains a little Vaseline petroleum jelly, turpentine, camphor, menthol, wheat germ oil, or any other type of medication you want to use. (Practitioners of Russian folk medicine boil half a pound of pure alum in two gallons of water.)
4. Pour the boiling hot water into the bucket, place the board over the top of the bucket, and then sit on the hole so that the steam will bathe your hemorrhoids.
5. After sitting on the bucket for about half an hour, pat the hemorrhoids dry with gauze or a soft towel.

How to replace protruding internal hemorrhoids

Hemorrhoids up in the rectum often slip down through the anus where they are painfully squeezed. A cold compress placed against the protruding hemorrhoids will reduce their size so that they can be oiled and pushed back into the rectum. This is best accomplished while lying on your side or while on your knees and elbows. Resting head-down on a steeply inclined slant board will help drain the swollen veins after they're replaced.

How to Soothe the Painful Agony of an Anal Fissure

Susan A. felt a sharp, burning pain around her anus while she was straining to empty her bowels. Thereafter, each bowel movement caused a splitting pain that was followed by bleeding. "I feel as if I'm having a baby every time I go to the toilet," she said.

Susan had an anal fissure, which means that she had literally split the opening to her rectum during a forced bowel movement. Here's what she did under my instructions to speed recovery and get relief from pain:

1. Each night before bedtime, she injected two ounces of cod liver oil into her rectum to lubricate and soften her stool. If you prefer, you may use olive oil or mineral oil. It may be necessary to wear a "diaper" to catch the leaking oil.
2. Twice daily, she put on a rubber glove and inserted a finger into her rectum to dilate and relax the muscular ring around her bowel opening. She lubricated the finger with Vaseline petroleum jelly.
3. After each bowel movement, Susan washed out her rectum with a cupful of cool water, which she injected with a syringe. When pain was present, she followed this with a hot hip bath.
4. Just to make sure that there was no roughage in her diet to rake the painful area, she ate such low-residue (soft) foods as eggs, ground lean meat, fish, cottage cheese, milk, potatoes, soups, bananas, fruit juices, oatmeal, and strained vegetables. She ate small meals and included an agar supplement for the moisture-retaining bulk she needed to guard against constipation.

After only a few weeks, the painful tear in her rectum had healed.

How to Ease an "Itching Bottom"

James J. seemed a little embarrassed when I asked him what his problem was. "I have this itching around my anus," he said, "and it's about to drive me crazy. It frequently keeps me awake at night—and it gets worse during hot weather."

James J. had what doctors call *pruritis ani.* I recommended a low-residue diet (see the section on anal fissure, page 143) and told him to take the following steps after each bowel movement:

1. After using toilet tissue, clean the anus with water-moistened cotton pads.
2. Then squat down over a large pan of slightly warm water so that the anus (opening) can be bathed.
3. Use a soft towel to pat the anus dry while in a squatting position and then apply a good medicated powder or a little plain cornstarch. If there is any drainage from the rectum, plug it with a piece of powdered cotton.

At every opportunity, James assumed a nude knee-chest position (on his knees and forearms) so that circulating air could dry the soft, swollen skin around his anus. It's very important to keep the itching area *as dry as possible,* since moisture or perspiration can aggravate the condition.

These simple measures eventually resulted in a complete cure for James, and they didn't cost him a cent. They also spared him the embarrassment of seeking medical care for a highly personal condition.

Summary

1. The majority of headaches can be relieved by relaxing the muscles of the neck with moist heat, massage, and traction.
2. A cup of strong coffee, an ice bag applied to the head, or a bandage wrapped tightly around the head will very often relieve a throbbing vascular headache.
3. You can cure constipation by visiting the toilet regularly and by eating fruits, vegetables, and other moisture-retaining foods that are rich in cellulose.
4. If you must eliminate the roughage in your diet for medical reasons, you can supplement your diet with agar-agar or psyllium seed extract for moisture-retaining bulk.
5. Injecting olive oil into your rectum a couple of hours before going to the toilet or before taking an enema will help empty a clogged rectum.
6. A hot hip bath, hot compresses applied to the anus, or an anal steam bath will provide soothing relief for external hemorrhoids.

7. Hemorrhoids can be lubricated by injecting a couple ounces of olive oil, mineral oil, cod liver oil, or any vegetable oil into the rectum.

8. Apply a cold compress to protruding external hemorrhoids and then dab them with oil before pushing them back into the rectum.

9. The anus and the rectum can be cleaned by washing with a sponge filled with cold water and by injecting a cupful of cool water into the rectum.

10. You can relieve an itching anus by keeping it very clean and as dry as possible.

9

How to Relieve the Pain and Misery of Stomach Ulcers, Colitis and Other Digestive Troubles with Naturomatic Healing

Your ability to digest and absorb food is so important to your general health that you cannot afford to ignore digestive troubles, even if they aren't painful. Many disorders of the stomach and the intestines are, in fact, quite painful, and all are distressing and weakening. There is, however, something that you can do about all of them, as you'll learn in this chapter.

A Simple Home-Care Program for Peptic Ulcer

Lewis M. complained of a gnawing "hunger pain" in the pit of his stomach. "I have a burning, aching pain right here," he said, pointing to a spot on his upper abdomen just below his breast bone. "It goes away when I eat and then comes back a couple of hours later. I usually have to get up in the middle of the night to eat something to relieve the pain." A little thumb pressure over the painful spot revealed a tender area about the size of a silver dollar.

Lewis had a peptic ulcer. Although he had been feeling the pain for more than a year, he obtained complete relief after only two weeks of using simple, natural remedies.

How to relieve pain and promote healing of stomach ulcers by eating special foods

Since the pain of a stomach or duodenal ulcer is usually caused by the corrosive action of stomach acid on a raw spot inside the stomach or the intestine, the pain can be relieved by putting food into the stomach to absorb the acid. A high-protein meal consisting of broiled meat, fish, poultry, eggs, and milk provides the greatest relief for the longest period of time. A small meal every two hours is usually most effective, since it absorbs acid without overstimulating the stomach.

Pain between meals can usually be relieved by drinking a glass of milk or by eating something. Yogurt or cottage cheese, for example, will absorb stomach acid without contributing excess calories. *The ulcer will eventually heal if it can be spared contact with undiluted stomach acid for a few weeks.*

Drink more milk and go easy on alkalizers

When ulcers are acutely painful, it may be necessary to eat or drink something every hour or so for pain relief. Milk and crackers are a favorite and have proven to be effective. You should be careful, however, not to combine antacids or alkalizers with milk. Such a combination could result in the absorption of a form of calcium that may be deposited in the kidneys or in the soft tissues around the joints. Antacids should be used only between meals or when "hunger pains" occur and food is not available to neutralize the excess acid.

Tablets containing natural calcium carbonate will relieve stomach acidity, but they tend to cause constipation and loss of magnesium. Many health food stores now sell tablets containing magnesium trisilicate and other effective antacids that *combat* constipation.

Special advice for victims of obesity and hardened arteries

If you can't drink whole milk because you're overweight or because your blood cholesterol is too high, skim milk may do just as well. If you like, you can add corn oil to the milk to delay absorption and to coat the stomach. The protein in skim milk will neutralize stomach acid as effectively as whole milk, but when the milk contains a little fat it stays in the stomach longer for longer pain relief. Corn oil will give you this effect, along with the essential fatty acids you need for clean arteries.

How to make corn-oil milk

You can make corn-oil milk daily by mixing 1½ tablespoons of honey and one teaspoon of powdered egg white in 12 ounces of skim milk in a blender. While mixing at slow speed, pour in six tablespoons of corn oil. Then add 12 more ounces of skim milk. A banana may be added for flavor. A little powdered skim milk may be added for extra nourishment.

Milk substitutes for allergy victims

If you are allergic to fresh cow's milk, use cultured milk, canned evaporated milk, or goat's milk. If you can't drink any type of milk or use milk products, you can snack on creamy cereals, cornstarch pudding, soft-boiled eggs, or Jello.

Soy milk is rich in protein, and may be useful in absorbing stomach acid. Blend one cup of full-fat soy flour and one-third of a cup of calcium lactate with one quart of water. Honey may be added for sweetening, and one egg white may be added for its antacid effect.

How to mix an effective household alkalizer

Ordinary household sodium bicarbonate is an effective antacid that will quickly relieve the pain of a stomach ulcer by neutralizing stomach acid. An overdose, however, can cause an "acid rebound," in which the stomach reacts by producing even more acid to overcome the alkalizing effect of the soda. So use as little as possible—and only when necessary to relieve pain.

Dip up just enough sodium bicarbonate to cover the tip of a spoon and stir it into a glass of cool water. Sip the water slowly so that you won't neutralize too much acid at one time. If you like, you may add two or three drops of essence of peppermint to the solution to help overcome the gas that's created by mixing acid and alkali in the stomach. A banana or a little creamy cereal containing a teaspoonful of fruit pectin, eaten one-half hour after taking soda, will absorb any acid rebound.

Remember that absorption of sodium bicarbonate into the system can cause illness from alkalosis if used excessively, so make *food* your first choice when it's available. Commercial antacids are not absorbed by the body, but they may have constipating or laxative effects.

Note: Many people have digestive troubles because they do not have enough acid in their stomach. There are, for example, many elderly persons who must take hydrochloric acid tablets with their meals in order to be able to digest their food and to absorb certain vitamins and minerals. You shouldn't take any kind of alkalizer if you don't have all the symptoms of a stomach ulcer.

How to make potato and cabbage alkalizers

Some healers maintain that the juice of raw white potatoes or cabbage has a healing, alkalizing effect on stomach ulcers. A juicer can be used to extract the juices from the fibers of these vegetables. Cabbage may be put through a meat grinder and then be squeezed in a cloth sack to press out the juice. A little vegetable oil added to the juice will delay its absorption in your stomach and prolong its effects.

Drink about a quart of cabbage juice each day, a glassful at a time—or six four-ounce glasses daily.

Special note! Recent research has revealed that cabbage juice contains Vitamin U, which has a healing effect on ulcers.

How to relieve stomach pain
with an ice bag

An ice bag applied to the portion of the spine between the shoulder blades, or to the abdomen just above the navel, will reduce the secretion of stomach acid and relieve a painful ulcer. When the ulcer is on the back wall of the stomach, the pain may radiate back into the spine. When this happens, place the ice bag over the portion of the spine where you feel the pain. The cold will numb the nerve fibers and short-circuit the pain reflex; thus yielding desired relief.

How to eat so that a stomach ulcer
can heal itself

An ulcer patient should try to eat as normal a diet as possible if he finds that he can eat the basic natural foods without any difficulty. Some doctors now tell their ulcer patients to eat anything that seems to agree with them. When some of the basic foods do seem to cause pain or bleeding from an ulcer, it may be necessary to eat foods that do not contain any roughage at all for a few days. Cream of wheat, gelatin, mashed potatoes, rice, eggs, cooked fruits, and vegetables that have been strained, bananas, diluted fruit juices, broiled meat or fish, cottage cheese, and milk, for example, are often recommended. A natural vitamin supplement containing vitamins A and C will speed healing. Most ulcer diets are deficient in Vitamin C.

Foods to avoid. When your ulcer is giving you trouble, you may have to avoid fried or spicy foods, carbonated beverages, coffee, alcohol, tobacco, raw vegetables, and coarse breads and cereals that may "scratch" an ulcer.

Soups, especially meat broths, should be avoided, since they stimulate the production of stomach acid without neutralizing the acid. The soups may, in fact, leave the stomach so rapidly that they leave an excess supply of gastric juice behind which can irritate the stomach.

How to make ulcer-healing
cream soups

If you must eat soup because of oral or dental problems, eat vegetable-type *cream soups* that contain milk. Puree your vegetables and then boil them in a cream sauce. One cup of milk or cream sauce to each one-half cup of vegetable puree should be about right.

Vegetables may also be pureed by steaming them and then pressing them through a fine sieve—or you may liquefy them in an electric blender. As soon as whole food can be tolerated, however, you should gradually work your way back to a normal diet. Begin by simply mashing your fruits and vegetables.

How to relieve constipation caused
by an ulcer diet

If you must follow a soft diet for very long, you may begin to suffer from constipation. So it might be a good idea to add a little agar or psyllium seed extract to your diet for non-irritating moisture-retaining bulk. Many doctors prescribe milk of magnesia as a bedtime medication, since it is both an antacid and a laxative. Some people find that a glass of milk and honey at bedtime will stimulate a morning bowel movement.

If you do become constipated, use some of the enema techniques described in Chapter 8. Return to a normal diet as soon as possible. Cooked fruits and vegetables should stimulate your bowels without irritating them. Keep an eye on your stools. If your ulcer should start bleeding again, your stools will become black resembling coffee grounds. This may mean that some of the foods you are eating are too coarse.

How to cure ulcers by relieving
emotional stress

It's now well-known that emotional stress and nervous tension can cause or aggravate ulcers. "Nervous" adrenal glands flood the body with certain hormones, which in turn flood the stomach with acid. Every doctor knows that the ulcers of an arthritic patient become worse when he is treated with cortisone and other adrenal gland hormones.

Be sure to study the tension-relieving techniques described in Chapter 3. Several days of complete rest are sometimes necessary to relieve the emotional stress that aggravates ulcers. This means *complete freedom from all cares and responsibilities.*

How to Relieve Indigestion Caused by Stomach Acid Deficiency

Jesse G. complained of "sour stomach," loss of appetite, and abdominal discomfort. "I've tried alkalizers," he said, "but they don't seem to help. In fact, I believe they make me worse. I belch up a sour taste, and I sometimes vomit."

Unlike Lewis M., who complained of stomach pain caused by an excessive amount of stomach acid, Jesse G. was suffering from *achylia gastrica,* which means that there was not enough acid in his stomach to digest his food. When he took alkalizers after a big meal, he triggered gas formation and vomiting by neutralizing what little acid there was in his stomach. *The addition of hydrochloric acid to his diet relieved his symptoms.*

You should never take an alkalizer just because you have overeaten. When your stomach is full, you need *more* rather than less stomach acid.

How to improve your digestion with acids and enzymes

If you have symptoms of hydrochloric acid deficiency, ask your druggist for a bottle of *dilute hydrochloric acid. Important:* Tell him it's for your indigestion. Mix one teaspoonful in half a glass of water and sip it through a glass straw during each meal. It's important to use a straw so that the acid won't erode your teeth.

You might prefer to take *glutamic hydrochloric acid tablets* with your meals. These tablets can be purchased in health food stores as well as in drug stores.

Apple cider or *lemon juice solutions* can sometimes be used in a pinch. Put a couple teaspoons of either in a glass of water and sip with your meals.

Pineapple and *papaya* contain enzymes that aid digestion. You can eat the fruit with meals or purchase the enzymes in health food stores.

Some of my patients with digestive troubles of unknown origin report that tablets containing *digestive enzymes and ox bile* are helpful.

Note: Hydrochloric acid deficiency is not uncommon in persons over 50 years of age. This deficiency is always present in persons who are suffering from pernicious anemia.

Hints for Relieving Ordinary Indigestion

If you suffer from indigestion that does not fit into any particular classification, there are a variety of everyday measures that you may employ to relieve your distress.

Don't rush your meals!

Always allow at least one hour for each meal. Chew your foods slowly, making sure that every particle of food is crushed by your teeth. Eat in quiet, pleasant surroundings, and then *relax* after eating. Rapid eating and inadequate chewing of food causes you to swallow air and bolt your food, which can lead to stomach cramps and intestinal gas.

A busy mechanic who was plagued by "indigestion" confessed that he rarely took more than 15 minutes to gulp down a couple of sandwiches and a cup of coffee at noon. When he hired a helper and started taking a whole hour for lunch, his digestive troubles disappeared. "I thought all the time that there was something seriously wrong with my stomach. I've spent a fortune on doctors, and I was planning to go to a big clinic for a checkup. But I'm all right now."

Quit smoking before dinner—
and go easy on coffee

If you must smoke cigarettes, don't smoke immediately before a meal. Smoking slows down the muscular waves (peristaltic action) in your stomach and intestines and delays the emptying of your stomach. This may allow cramps and unpleasant fermentation to develop.

Excessive coffee drinking can also contribute to indigestion. If you drink a lot of coffee, use the type that doesn't contain caffeine.

Eliminate grease and fat— and eat fresh, natural foods

The less greasy or fatty foods you eat, the better. Too much fat in your diet inhibits digestion and delays emptying of your stomach. If you happen to have gall bladder trouble, a greasy diet will cause nausea and other symptoms of illness. Eat fresh, natural foods that are not fried or soaked in grease.

Get your teeth in shape

If you have bad teeth—or no teeth at all—and you cannot chew your food properly, see your dentist (and read Chapter 10). Lumpy, unchewed foods in your stomach can cause nausea, heart burn, cramps, and other symptoms of indigestion.

Lucille R. started suffering from indigestion after having only three of her teeth extracted. "I've never had trouble with my digestion before," she said. "I've had all kinds of X-rays made and nothing seems to be wrong." When she was fitted with dental bridges and could once again chew her food properly, her digestion returned to normal.

Go easy on gas-forming foods—and declare war on gas-forming bacteria

Gas that can be expelled by belching is usually only swallowed air. Gas pains in the lower abdomen, however, may be caused by such gas-forming foods as cucumbers, radishes, beans, cabbage, turnips, onions, raw apples, and cauliflower. Most people are aware that certain foods give them "gas." Raw salads or milk, for example, may disturb one person and not another.

Putrefaction of foods, particularly protein, in the lower intestinal tract, can form foul-smelling gas. This can very often be relieved by including yogurt or cultured acidophilus milk in your diet to increase the number of lactobacillus (bacteria) in your colon. These helpful bacteria destroy putrefactive bacteria by producing lactic acid. Your druggist or health food store usually has a line of these cultures to combat putrefaction in your system.

How to take a special enema
to relieve gas pressure

If you are bothered constantly by intestinal gas or flatulence, you may be able to relieve gas pains with a *carminative enema.* Mix two teaspoons of spirits of peppermint into a quart of warm water and use the enema technique described in Chapter 8. Or inject one of the following formulas into your lower bowel: eight ounces of molasses mixed with eight ounces of warm milk; one-half ounce of turpentine mixed with six ounces of warm olive oil; or eight ounces each of sugar and sodium bicarbonate mixed with eight ounces of water. (Use a *fluid measuring cup* to measure out eight ounces of sugar and eight ounces of soda, and then mix both into eight ounces of warm water. Stir until the sugar and soda dissolve to make a soupy solution.)

Warning: If you use the turpentine and olive oil formula, you should take a cleansing, plain-water enema one-half to one hour later.

How to relieve abdominal pain
with hot packs

A hot pack placed over the abdomen will relieve gas pain and intestinal spasm. You may use a flaxseed poultice or a simple hot fomentation (see Chapter 7). A few drops of turpentine are sometimes added to the water used in making an abdominal fomentation. Be careful, however, not to use so much turpentine that you blister your skin.

Warning: Before placing any type of heat on your abdomen,

you must make sure that you don't have appendicitis or an intestinal infection. If you have a fever, or if pressure on the lower right side of your abdomen causes pain, your appendix may be inflamed, which means that it would be best to use a cold pack.

Measures for Coping with Simple Diarrhea

When diarrhea that is not caused by disease or infection occurs, there are several things that you can do to relieve your discomfort.

Clean your intestine
with a 24-hour fast

When your bowels suddenly begin "running off," it might be a good idea to fast for at least one day so that your intestinal tract will have a chance to clean out the toxin or irritant.

Check diarrhea with
buttermilk and bananas

Cultured buttermilk, which is rich in lactic acid and friendly bacteria, is sometimes recommended for persistent diarrhea. Bananas, which contain pectin that helps absorb and eliminate poisons, may also be of value in ending diarrhea.

How to correct dehydration
caused by diarrhea

Because of the danger of dehydration from chronic diarrhea, you should begin drinking water or juices as soon as your stomach will tolerate them. Salty soups or broths will temporarily help your body absorb and hold water.

A water-retention enema. If you're unable to retain liquids because of nausea, you can inject several ounces of warm water into your rectum several times a day. If you'll hold the water as long as you can before releasing it, your body will absorb enough of the water to keep you from "drying out." Plain water enemas will also help wash out residual poisons that may be prolonging the diarrhea.

Note: Prolonged or severe diarrhea that is accompanied by abdominal cramps, fever, and foamy, bloody stools should be brought to the attention of a physician.

Warning: milk causes diarrhea in some people

Although milk is prescribed frequently in the treatment of ulcers and other stomach disorders, the sugar or lactose in milk can cause diarrhea in some people. There are some people, for example, who lack an enzyme needed to digest and absorb milk sugar. When this is the case, the lactose passes down into the lower intestine where it stimulates bacterial action that causes excessive gas or diarrhea. You can test your sensitivity to milk by taking a dose of pure lactose.

Some of my patients who are sensitive to milk report that when they need a natural laxative, they either drink milk or take pure lactose.

Richard B. experienced daily gas pains and abdominal cramps until he replaced his usual milk and cereal breakfast with fresh fruit, lean meat, eggs, and other foods that did not contain milk. "A little honey in hot oatmeal is a good substitute for dry cereal and milk," he said.

Fermented milk products are low in lactose. If you find that you cannot tolerate lactose, you can switch to yogurt, buttermilk, or cottage cheese for your milk nutrients. These mild products— and cheeses of all types—are low in lactose because of bacterial action that has converted the lactose to lactic acid. Yogurt cultured with acidophilus bacteria is particularly helpful in normalizing intestinal function.

How to Cope with Colitis and Diverticulitis

Chronic or recurring diarrhea can often be traced to colon trouble. Colitis and diverticulitis are two common colon disorders that require a lot of home care.

A physician should be consulted when diarrhea persists unrelieved. Tumors or polyps in the colon are sometimes a cause of chronic diarrhea.

Colitis, food, and mind power

Diarrhea caused by colitis or inflammation of the lower bowel is very often the result of emotional stress. Whenever this is the case, rest and freedom from stress may be the only cure. Fluids and juices, cooked fruits and vegetables, broiled meats, eggs, cheeses, and other vitamin-rich, non-irritating *natural* foods should be a part of the diet. Refined carbohydrates should be completely eliminated. Some doctors recommend a low-carbohydrate diet to reduce intestinal fermentation. It may occasionally be necessary to strain or puree fruits and vegetables until the diarrhea subsides.

How to handle an inflamed, constipated colon

When colitis is accompanied by constipation that is characterized by dry, hard, mucus-covered stools, a non-irritating diet along with measures to combat constipation (see Chapter 8) may be helpful. Foods that are rich in roughage, however, such as corn, nuts, whole wheat, and raw vegetables should be avoided until intestinal spasms subside. Otherwise, irritation of an already inflamed colon triggers painful spasm that blocks the bowels.

Hot applications applied to the abdomen will relieve pain and cramps.

In many cases, a period of spasm and constipation will be followed by diarrhea. The diarrhea will not return if the constipation is corrected and the colitis is relieved.

The cause and cure of diverticulitis

More than one-third of all Americans over 40 years of age have tiny pouches or "diverticula" on the walls of their colon. When these pouches become clogged and inflamed, painful abdominal cramps—usually in the lower left portion of the abdomen—occur along with constipation or diarrhea.

Sixty-eight-year-old Eva H., for example, experienced abdominal cramps and constipation after eating a batch of fresh strawberries. This was followed a few days later by diarrhea. X-ray examination revealed the presence of numerous small pouches on the lower portion of her colon. Her doctor prescribed a "soft" diet made up largely of white-flour products and starches, which did not seem to help much.

It's generally accepted that food roughage must be reduced in the care of diverticulitis. A complete lack of vegetable fibers, however, may only allow sticky waste to pack itself into tiny crevices and pouches. When Eva included cooked fruits and vegetables in her diet, her abdominal cramps disappeared and her bowels moved normally.

Some doctors now believe that the cellulose provided by fruits and vegetables will help *clean* rather than clog intestinal pouches. An article in the May 22, 1971, *British Medical Journal,* for example, states that diverticulosis, or the formation of colon pouches, appears to be *caused* by refined carbohydrates that clog and stretch the colon. If you don't already have colon trouble, be sure to eat plenty of fresh fruits and vegetables each day. The more vegetable fiber there is in your diet, the healthier your colon will be.

How to eat to relieve diverticulitis

Bran, grain and seed husks, fruit and vegetable seeds, fruit skins, spices, and other grainy forms of roughage may irritate inflamed intestinal pouches and should be eliminated.

Meat, eggs, milk, cheeses, cooked fruits and vegetables, fruit and vegetable juices, and other non-irritating *natural* foods should be a part of a soft diet until symptoms subside. Be careful not to eat fruits and vegetables containing seeds and husks, such as tomatoes and corn.

When constipation occurs, it's all right to take a cleansing enema, but you should not take laxatives.

If you find it necessary to eliminate all fruits and vegetables during an acute attack of diverticulitis, you should include a little agar or psyllium seed extract in your diet for its bulk and laxative effects. As soon as symptoms permit, however, you should gradually work your way back to cooked fruits and vegetables and then to fresh fruits and salads. You need cellulose to keep your colon open and clean. And remember that cellulose retains moisture and helps the growth of the bacteria you need to prevent putrefaction in your colon.

Summary

1. Frequent, small meals of protein-rich foods will relieve the pain of a stomach ulcer by absorbing stomach acid.
2. Constipation caused by an ulcer diet can be relieved with enemas and agar or psyllium seed supplements.
3. A thimbleful of baking soda mixed into a glass of water and sipped slowly will relieve ulcer pain by neutralizing stomach acid.
4. Raw cabbage juice and pureed raw Idaho potatoes have a healing, alkalizing effect on stomach ulcers.
5. Sour stomach and indigestion caused by a *deficiency* of stomach acid can be relieved by sipping dilute hydrochloric acid and water with meals.
6. Hot packs placed over the abdomen will relieve pain caused by gas and intestinal spasm. (Be careful that the condition is not appendicitis: other measures are necessary if that is the case.)
7. Simple diarrhea can usually be relieved with a one-day fast, cultured buttermilk, and bananas.
8. Yogurt or cultured milk containing lactobacillus acidophilus will produce the lactic acid you need to kill putrefactive, gas-forming bacteria in your colon.
9. An inflamed colon, characterized by cramps with constipation or diarrhea, should be protected from excessive roughage with a soft diet made up of *natural* foods.
10. Refined carbohydrates clog the colon and produce constipation, diverticulosis, and spasm, whereas fresh fruits and vegetables containing cellulose keep the colon clean and open.

10

How to Care for Your Teeth, Gums, Bones and Joints with Naturomatic Healing Methods

Most people think of the teeth and the bones as being indestructible. The skeletal remains of humans and animals certainly seem to indicate that this might be so. The truth is, however, that in a living body there is a constant exchange of wastes and nutrients to maintain the strength and soundness of both the teeth and the bones. When there is a nutritional deficiency in the body, or when stresses are abnormal, even the best teeth and the hardest bones will begin to deteriorate—far more rapidly in a living body than in a corpse. This is why natural remedies for disorders of the bones and the teeth must provide nutrients as well as relieve pain. You'll learn about these remedies in this chapter, and what you learn will provide benefits that will last a lifetime.

How to Stop the Progress of Pyorrhea and Other Gum Diseases

No matter how well you care for your teeth, you won't be able to keep them if you don't take care of your gums. In persons over 40 years of age, *gum disease accounts for more lost teeth than all other factors combined.* Three out of every four Americans suffer from gum trouble that dentists call periodontal disease. Almost

100 percent of all Americans over the age of 65 have gum disease! So it's likely that *all* of us will have to contend with gum trouble sooner or later. The gums simply recede and become detached from the teeth, allowing food particles, bacteria, and mineral deposits to accumulate under the edges of the gums. This leads to infection that erodes the attaching membranes and the roots of the teeth. The teeth then become loose and may actually fall out if the infection isn't stopped.

How to recognize the early warning signs of gum disease

Slight bleeding from your gums while you are brushing your teeth may mean that you are developing gum disease. If your gums are red and puffy and some of your teeth seem to be loose in their sockets, you may already have pyorrhea or periodontal disease. See your dentist as soon as possible, and begin a self-help program immediately. Failure to help yourself, even if you are under the care of a dentist, could result in loss of your teeth.

Larry C. was only 38 years of age when he first began to suffer from "gum boils." He had also noticed that his gums would bleed when he brushed his teeth. "I have good teeth," he insisted. "I have only two or three fillings, and I have no cavities. Furthermore, I brush my teeth every day." Five years later, Larry still had no cavities, but his teeth had gotten so loose that many of them had to be pulled. He was suddenly a dental cripple, no longer able to eat normally. Had he taken proper care of his gums with simple home remedies, he could have saved his teeth.

Thelma V. took immediate action when she noticed that some of her teeth were loose. After having her teeth cleaned by a dentist, she started a self-help program that required daily care for her gums and her teeth. After only a few months, her teeth tightened normally and the color of her gums changed from an angry red to a normal pink color.

Even if you do not now have any apparent gum trouble, you should devote as much attention to your gums as to your teeth. In fact, it's absolutely necessary that you do so if you want to keep your teeth!

Home care for your teeth and gums

Observe these rules every day of your life for good teeth and healthy gums:

1. *Brush your teeth after each meal.* Select a brush that has soft bristles. Brush back and forth with short strokes, across the teeth at the gum margin, so that the bristles will slip up under the edge of the gum.

To brush the back of the front teeth, hold your brush in a vertical position and use up-and-down strokes.

Be sure to brush every gum margin and every tooth on both sides. You can buy a red food dye in the form of "discoloring wafers" that can be used to stain the deposits on your teeth. When you have brushed away all the stains, you'll know that you have cleaned your teeth adequately.

A simple household cleaner for your teeth. A teaspoonful of salt or sodium bicarbonate in a glass of warm water, used with a tooth brush, will clean your teeth as effectively as any toothpaste. Plain sodium bicarbonate can be used to clean teeth that are coated with sticky plaque or bacterial waste.

2. *Clean between your teeth and under the edge of your gums with dental floss.* Use the unwaxed variety so that it won't be too slippery to rake deposits off your teeth. Slide the floss up and down against one side of a tooth until the floss squeaks. Move the floss as far up under the edge of the gum as you can without causing pain. (There is a slight crevice under the margin of the healthy gum. This crevice deepens considerably in gum disease.) Remember that you must clean under the edges of the gum on *both sides* of each tooth.

Be careful not to cut your gum with the floss. When two teeth are close together, it may be necessary to work the floss back and forth until it slips through a tight spot.

It takes more than 24 hours for hard deposits to form on your teeth, so it may not be necessary to use dental floss more often than once daily. If you have large pockets under the edges of your gums, however, you may have to use the floss after each meal to remove food particles that might give off odors from fermentation or decomposition.*

---

*Jets of water from an oral irrigating appliance, available in drug stores, will clean out deep gum pockets.

Note: Food deposits that are only a day or two old can be removed with floss or a tooth brush, but tartar or calculus that forms under the gum margins must be removed by a dentist.

3. *Don't eat between meals.* Once you have eaten and you have cleaned your teeth and gums, you should not eat between meals and risk trapping food particles in gum pockets. Starches and sweets, especially, ferment quickly and serve as food for acid-forming bacteria that are constantly "waiting in the wings" for the nourishment they need to feed the infection that erodes the bone around the roots of your teeth.

Bacterial activity in gum pockets may cause bad breath many months before infection causes swelling or an abscess. If your breath has a bad odor, be sure to have your gums examined. If you have gum pockets, your bad breath will persist in spite of regular brushing, especially if you eat between meals. In some cases, it may be necessary for a periodontist, a dentist specializing in gum surgery, to cut away the pockets deep beneath your gums.

If you must eat between meals, you should eat apples, carrots, celery, and other fresh fruits and vegetables. Natural foods that are rich in cellulose will *clean* your teeth as well as provide exercise for your teeth and your gums.

4. *Use interdental stimulators between meals.* When you do eat between meals and you aren't able to brush your teeth or use dental floss, you can clean your teeth with interdental stimulators. These are soft toothpick-like strips of balsa wood that can be pressed between the teeth and against the gum margin. They won't damage the teeth or the gums as a hardwood toothpick might do.

You can purchase interdental stimulators in matchbox size containers in any drug store. Carry a package in your pocket, or keep one in your desk drawer.

Note: No matter what method you use to clean your teeth, you should rinse your teeth with water after eating.

5. *Don't clench your teeth.* Many nervous people who are constantly clenching or grinding their teeth actually loosen their teeth by jamming them into their sockets. And if the teeth don't fit together as they should, the loosening may be so rapid that soreness and swelling result, with progressive loss of bone around the roots of the teeth. Many people have developed gum disease and lost teeth because of habitual teeth clenching.

Teeth grinding during the night is usually due to emotional tension, but it may also be a sign of nutritional deficiency.

How to improve the health of your teeth and gums with good nutrition

It is known that a Vitamin C deficiency causes bleeding gums and loosens teeth. Few people these days are so deficient in Vitamin C that they show classic signs of scurvy, but enough of us are deficient in this important vitamin to suffer from tender gums. If you have any kind of gum trouble, you should eat plenty of fresh fruits and vegetables and take a natural Vitamin C supplement.

Vitamin A is also essential for healthy gums and for fighting infection. If you must restrict animal fat in your diet because of hardened arteries or high blood pressure, increase your intake of yellow vegetables and take a little fish liver oil.

A calcium or Vitamin D deficiency can result in loss of bone around the roots of the teeth. Bone meal tablets enriched with Vitamin D will supply all the vitamins and minerals your body needs to build bone.

Protein is essential for the supporting tissues of the teeth. The tough fibers that hold the teeth in their bony sockets, for example, must be sustained by plenty of protein and Vitamin C.

A deficiency of almost any vitamin or mineral may contribute to the development of gum disease or tooth decay—even in the cleanest mouth. So it's important to make sure that your diet is well balanced with fresh, natural foods.

Quit eating sugar and refined starches! In addition to feeding bacteria that cause tooth decay and gum infection, refined sugars and starches may trigger the development of diabetes, a disease in which sugar accumulates in the blood. Gum infections are difficult or impossible to control when sugar-rich blood is constantly feeding the infection from within.

First Aid for a Toothache and an Abscess

A wad of cotton soaked with oil of clove and packed into the cavity of an aching tooth will usually result in quick relief from pain. If that doesn't help, apply an ice bag to the jaw or place a piece of ice in your mouth. When the pulp inside a tooth is infected or inflamed, a cold mouthwash will relieve the pain. Dipping a finger in whiskey and then using the finger to massage the gum around a troublesome tooth will often provide relief.

When there is an infection or an abscess, resulting in a swollen jaw, wrap a couple of ice cubes in a wash cloth and apply it over the swollen area for ten to fifteen minutes at a time, as many times as necessary to relieve the pain. Rinse the mouth frequently with warm, salty water to help open and drain the abscess. A half-teaspoon of salt in each glass of water will do.

How to Replace a Dislocated Jaw

Sandra K. was watching a boring TV movie when she yawned and snapped her jaw out of place. Unable to speak with her mouth locked in a wide-open position, she could only grunt and wave her arms in communicating her distress. Fortunately, her husband knew what to do. He unlocked her jaw with a simple manipulation that he had read about in a trainer's manual.

Once a jaw dislocates, it's very likely to happen again. So it might be a good idea to keep these instructions handy for first aid purposes and to save the expense of hospital emergency calls.

1. Wrap both of your thumbs with a thick layer of gauze and then tape them with plain adhesive tape to protect them from injury.
2. Sit the victim down on a low stool in front of you and then grip his jaws so that your thumbs rest on top of his lower back teeth on each side.
3. Press down with your thumbs—with considerable force—until the jaw ligaments begin to stretch. Then add a little backward pressure. This will force the jaw to slide over a ridge and back into its shallow socket.

How to Restore Strength to Aching, Fragile Bones

A 75-year-old widow was pushing against a piano when she suddenly felt a pain in her back just above her waist. X-ray examination revealed a compression fracture of one of her verte-brae.

Bessie D., sixty-three, fractured three ribs when she reached from the front seat of her car to the back seat for a package. A year later, she sneezed and fractured two ribs!

Clinton P., a 72-year-old retired accountant, discovered that he had two collapsed vertebrae in his lower back during a routine X-ray examination for backache.

All of these people had one thing in common: their bones were porous and brittle from lack of adequate minerals. In addition to suffering from aching bones and joints, all were subject to fractures in the performance of simple, everyday activities. The measures they took to rebuild their bones should be a part of your own program to relieve aches and pains that stem from deep within your bones.

The older you become, the greater the tendency for your bones to lose calcium. Women past the age of 50, or women who have had their ovaries removed, frequently develop brittle bones or osteoporosis that results from a hormone deficiency. The "dowager's hump," which is a hump back that frequently develops in women past middle age, is usually the result of osteoporosis or calcium deficiency. The softened vertebrae simply become com-pressed under the weight of the body and the pull of gravity.

Hip fractures, which are so common among elderly women, are usually also the result of a mineral deficiency. In some cases, a hip will fracture spontaneously while walking or climbing stairs. The fall that results is often falsely believed to be the cause of the fracture.

An increased intake of calcium in the years past middle age will help overcome the tendency of the bones to crumble.

How to get the vitamins and minerals
you need to rebuild weak bones

Your body must have calcium, phosphorus, Vitamin D, mag-nesium, and protein to build bones. If any one of these elements is missing, your bones will be soft or brittle.

Milk and milk products (such as cottage cheese) are the best food sources of *calcium*. Green leafy vegetables are fairly rich in calcium, but spinach, beet greens, chard, and rhubarb contain oxalic acid, which interferes with the absorption of calcium.

Protein foods of animal origin are the best sources of *protein,* and they supply the *phosphorus* you need to utilize calcium. Most vegetables contain some protein, but all of them, with the exception of soy beans, are deficient in some of the amino acids your body needs to utilize the protein.*

Sunlight and fish liver oil are the best sources of *Vitamin D.* You can, however, buy milk that has been enriched with Vitamin D.

Dolomite, which is powdered limestone taken from the earth, is a good source of *magnesium.* Foods containing protein usually also contain magnesium, but nuts, peas and beans, and whole grain cereals are probably the best food sources.

You should, of course, increase your intake of natural foods containing bone-building ingredients. If you already have osteoporosis or soft bones, you should supplement your diet with the vitamins and minerals your body needs to build bone rapidly. *Bone meal* enriched with Vitamin D contains all the essential bone-building elements. If you bake your own bread, you might want to mix a little bone meal in with the flour, but remember that the phytic acid in wheat tends to interfere with the absorption of calcium.

Your stomach needs acid to absorb calcium

If you have weak bones in spite of eating properly, your stomach may not be secreting the hydrochloric acid it needs to absorb calcium. You can solve this problem by taking glutamic hydrochloric acid tablets with your meals.

Taking alkalizers or antacids can interfere with the absorption of calcium by neutralizing stomach acid. So don't get into the habit of taking combinations of aspirin and alkalizers for headache, colds, upset stomach, and other minor ailments.

If you have gall bladder trouble, inadequate digestion of fat

---

*Persons who are on a heavy meat diet need extra calcium—more than 800 milligrams a day—to balance the phosphorus supplied by the meat. Otherwise, a calcium deficiency will develop.

might interfere with absorption of fat-soluble Vitamin D, which you must have to use calcium in building bones. Tablets containing ox bile can be added to meals for better digestion. A little olive oil or vegetable oil on a raw salad before each meal will stimulate the function of the gall bladder.

Fifty-year-old Dolly C. had complained of backache and aching joints for at least two years before she learned that her bones were deficient in calcium. Her aches and pains disappeared after she supplemented her diet with glutamic hydrochloric acid and bone-building vitamins and minerals. "Keep taking those supplements," I told her, "and you won't have to worry about a dowager's hump or a broken hip in the years to come."

How to speed the healing of a fracture

If you ever suffer the misfortune of a broken bone, you can speed your recovery by observing these simple rules:

1. *Mix a little bone meal in homemade bread,* milk, soup, meat loaf, and other foods—or take some bone meal tablets three times daily.
2. *Get out into the sunlight some each day.* The action of the sun's rays on the skin forms Vitamin D that is absorbed by the body. Many people who suffer a hip or leg fracture are confined to bed for several weeks without any exposure to the sun. If they aren't given a Vitamin D supplement, they may not be able to use calcium effectively because of a Vitamin D deficiency.

If you're ever confined to bed, especially for a fracture, try to expose more than just your face to the sun's rays for a few minutes each day. You don't have to stay out long enough to get a tan, and you should certainly try to avoid a sunburn.

There are many city workers who live and work in the shade of gigantic skyscrapers and who spend most of their life under a ceiling of smoke and smog. It's no wonder that some of them suffer from brittle and porous bones. Bone-building ultraviolet rays will filter through light fog and haze, but not through heavy air pollution.

3. *Be as active as possible.* Bones become stronger and thicker when they are subjected to weight bearing and muscular contraction. They become weak and thin when they are *not* subjected to stress. There are many old people, for example, who have brittle bones simply because they are inactive.

No matter how good your diet may be, your bones will lose calcium if you don't get any exercise. Even the astronauts must exercise during short space journeys in order to keep the calcium in their bones. Living bone will store only enough calcium to meet the existing stresses. When there is prolonged inactivity, the kidneys begin excreting the calcium released by the bones.

Isometric contraction for broken limbs. When you have a broken bone, your activities will, of necessity, be limited. But you may be able to maintain the strength of the injured bone—and even speed its healing—by contracting the involved muscles as soon as you're able to do so without pain. If a splint or cast prevents joint movement, just "set" or tense the muscles isometrically—that is, without attempting to move the joints.

Summary

1. Always clean your teeth after eating so that food particles won't feed the bacteria that contribute to tooth decay and gum infection.
2. Stain your teeth with "discoloring wafers" and then brush them to see if you brush away all the stained food particles.
3. Clean between your teeth and under the edges of your gums with dental floss at least once every 24 hours.
4. A simple salt or soda solution used with a toothbrush will clean your teeth as effectively as any toothpaste.
5. Bad breath or bleeding gums may mean that you have periodontal disease, caused by pockets under the gum margins.
6. You can improve the health of your gums by taking Vitamin C and by eliminating the refined sugars and starches in your diet.
7. A wad of cotton soaked in oil of clove and stuffed into the cavity of a bad tooth will usually relieve a toothache.
8. Brittle, porous bones that ache and fracture easily must have

more calcium, along with phosphorus, Vitamin D, and magnesium.

9. Bone meal that has been enriched with Vitamin D contains all the elements your body needs to build and repair bones.

10. Inactivity weakens bones, while the stress of weight bearing and muscular contraction *strengthens* bones.

11

How to Treat Simple Skin Disorders with Naturomatic Healing

"A skin specialist has the best practice of all," a wit once said. "His patients never die, and they never get well."

Few diseases are as difficult to diagnose and treat as skin ailments. Hundreds of different disorders of the skin, all with different causes, closely resemble each other. Allergies, nutritional deficiencies, emotional stress, and other factors all have some effect on the skin. Almost without exception, however, *a chronic skin condition must be cured from within*—that is, the body must heal itself. This isn't possible without natural remedies that improve health and normalize body chemistry.

In this chapter, you'll learn how to handle some common and not-so-common skin disorders with home remedies that will fit right in with your health-building program.

How to Cope with Dry Skin

Persons who are born with an insufficient number of oil glands in their skin are lifelong victims of dry skin. This means that every day of their lives they must make an effort to protect their skin from excessive drying that leads to redness, itching, scaling, or chapping.

Go easy on using soap. Excessive use of soap will wash away the protective oil of the skin. Actually, the skin normally has an oily, acid coating that keeps it soft and pliable and protects it from infection. In addition to washing away the oil, alkaline soaps neutralize the skin acids and leave the skin vulnerable to infection by fungus or bacteria. So when you do use soap, select a mild, nearly neutral soap.

When soap seems to leave your skin too dry, rub your body with a little olive oil, or bathe in fresh water that contains a little olive oil and a few drops of lemon juice. Many older people who suffer from dry skin cannot use soap at all except on their hands, face, scalp, feet, and groin. *When the skin is very dry and deficient in oil, soap is not needed for cleaning.* A plain water bath followed by rubbing a little olive oil into the skin is all that's needed.

In the winter, when perspiration is diminished, the skin may become so dry that the use of soap results in "winter itch." So while it may be necessary to use a little soap during the summer, you may have to substitute an oil bath in the winter and use soap only on "dirty spots."

How Jennie cured a dry skin rash

One of my patients, Jennie T., was not aware that she had "dry skin" until she broke out in a peculiar rash that defied diagnosis and treatment. After a couple of years making the rounds of doctors' offices, she came to me for help. "I'm no skin specialist," I told her, "but it appears to me that you might be deficient in the essential fatty acids." I recommended Vitamin F and suggested that she put a couple tablespoons of safflower oil on a daily green salad and then rub a little olive oil on her skin after each bath. The results were amazing. In less than two weeks, her skin looked perfectly normal!

Simple natural remedies can often work wonders. And they never do any harm. So don't hesitate to try a remedy that sounds "too simple to be effective." Like Jennie T., you might spend hundreds of dollars and suffer needlessly while searching for a cure that is already available to you at home. I've seen many ailments respond to simple remedies that doctors have refused to consider.

How to Cope with Oily Skin

If you have oily skin, your skin-care program will be just the opposite of that recommended for victims of dry skin. Frequent use of soap and water will be needed to dissolve the oil that accumulates in the pores of the skin. *And the more oil there is on the skin, the stronger and more alkaline the soap should be.* The face, which is the oiliest part of the body, must sometimes be washed a couple of times a day to wash away the oil. The scalp, which is the second oiliest part of the body, must be washed with soap three or four times a week to wash away oil and dead skin that tends to cake together and form dandruff. If oily dandruff is allowed to accumulate on the scalp, bacteria may collect and start an infection.

Reducing your intake of sugar, starch, and fats will reduce oiliness in the skin.

How to Clean Skin Pores and Help Cure Acne

Many people who suffer from extremely oily skin also suffer from acne, a skin condition in which clogged oil glands become swollen and infected. Follow these simple suggestions to open clogged pores and to speed the healing of infected skin.

Wash frequently
with strongly alkaline soap

Some doctors suggest that acne victims use laundry soap (such as Octagon or Fels-Naptha) for its drying and degreasing effects, especially over the neck and shoulders. Use plenty of hot, soapy water so that the skin becomes so dry that it actually peels. Take a shower each morning and each evening, with as much face washing as possible between showers.

Press plugs out of pores

The application of hot, moist towels to the face after a hot, soapy shower will soften the oil plugs or "blackheads" so that they can be pressed out with light fingertip pressure. Or you can use a special "comedone expresser" that can be purchased in any drugstore. You shouldn't squeeze swollen or infected bumps, however, since that may only push the infection deeper into the tissues. After the pores have been cleaned out, rinse the skin with cold water and dab on a little alcohol. Do all of this at night just before you go to bed so that you won't have to expose your face to contamination by dust or perspiration. Freshly opened pores are easily infected during the first few hours after cleaning, so it might be a good idea to change pillow cases every time you clean your face.

Note: Touching acne bumps with the fingers during the day is a common cause of infection. When you're not bathing, *keep your hands off your face.*

It is important to watch your diet!

Don't eat refined or greasy foods. This means eliminating fried foods and white-sugar and white-flour products. Eat plenty of fresh fruits and vegetables. No candy, soft drinks, pastries, and foods of that type. If it's not a *natural* food, don't eat it! And that goes for foods containing chemical additives and preservatives.

If you find that your acne is aggravated by milk, eggs, wheat, nuts, chocolate, pork, cheese, bananas, tomatoes, onions, citrus fruits, or shell fish, eliminate the offending food from your diet.

Drugs containing bromides or iodides can aggravate acne. So can iodized salt. If you must use salt each day, buy the type that does not contain iodine, but make sure that you eat some type of seafood at least once a week.

Soften skin oil with Vitamin F

The soft or unsaturated fat (Vitamin F) found in vegetable oil may help to keep skin oil from clogging pores. Add about two tablespoons of cold-pressed corn oil, wheat germ oil, or safflower oil to a fresh, green salad each day.

Correct Vitamin A deficiency

It's well known that a Vitamin A deficiency can contribute to the development of acne. If you are unable to eat plenty of green and yellow vegetables each day, or if you are on a low-fat diet, you should supplement your diet with fish liver oil. If you take a Vitamin A capsule, about 25,000 units a day should be enough. Remember that excessive doses of Vitamin A over a long period of time can have toxic effects.

Expose your skin to ultraviolet rays

The ultraviolet rays of sunlight may speed the healing of acne by killing germs and peeling the skin. Remember, however, that sweating may aggravate acne by increasing the production of skin oil. For this reason, you might prefer to use an ultraviolet lamp in an air-conditioned room rather than sunbathe outdoors. You must be careful not to burn yourself when you use a lamp. There is no heat in ultraviolet rays, so there is no way to tell when you have had enough. Begin with only a few seconds exposure the first day and then increase the exposure from day to day if no painful reaction occurs. Always protect your eyes from ultraviolet rays. *Don't ever look directly into an ultraviolet lamp.* Cover your eyes with pads of moist cotton when the rays are directed toward your face.

How to Relieve an Itching Skin

There are many skin conditions that cause itching. No matter what the condition, however, there are some basic treatments that you can use to provide immediate relief from aggravating sleep-killing itch. Try all the various treatments and then decide for yourself which works best for you.

How to take a cornstarch bath

When a large portion of your body is "itching like mad," immersion of your body in a tub of cornstarch solution may give you the relief you're seeking.

Mix one pound of cornstarch with enough cold water to make a smooth paste. Then add hot water and boil the mixture down until it becomes thick. Mix the paste into a tub of warm water (about 100 degrees F.) and then soak in the water for 15 or 20 minutes. When you get out of the tub, pat your skin dry so that a thin film of starch will remain on your skin.

Oatmeal water treatment

Cook about three cups of oatmeal. Strain the oatmeal over a tub of warm water. Then wrap the oatmeal in a cloth bag so that it can be squeezed in the water to press out the creamy starch. While soaking your body in the water, pat your skin with the bag of oatmeal—or use the bag as a washcloth. Oatmeal water, without soap, has a cleansing effect on the skin.

You can purchase a special oatmeal powder in any drugstore for mixing in bath water. Simply wrapping a handful of oatmeal or bran in a cloth bag and squeezing it in your bath water will be adequate in some cases.

Sodium bicarbonate bath benefits

An alkaline bath is sometimes recommended for itchy skin. Mix two tablespoons of baking soda in a tub of water that has a comfortable temperature. Soak in the water until the itching subsides. Remember, however, that the skin is normally acid. So use an alkaline bath only when it seems to relieve itching.

A paste made up of sodium bicarbonate and water can be applied over small areas of the body.

How to relieve itching
with hot cloths

It's well known that sweating will increase most forms of itching. Yet, recent research has shown that very hot water—120 to 130 degrees Fahrenheit— applied to the skin with a wash cloth will relieve intense itching over small areas. (Remember that bath water should not be hotter than 112 degrees.)

If the hot cloth doesn't seem to help, try patting the itchy spots with a bag of boiled cornstarch or cooked oatmeal or with a baking soda paste.

How to Relieve an Itchy Scalp with an Egg Shampoo

If you have an itchy scalp because of an allergy to soap, you might want to take an egg shampoo. Just beat three eggs, wet your head with water, and then "wash" your scalp with the eggs. Finish with a vinegar rinse and a final fresh-water rinse. Use the shampoo once a week for at least a month, or until the allergy subsides.

How to Relieve Itching Insect Bites

An itchy flea or mosquito bite is not a serious condition—until it begins to interfere with your sleep. When this happens, you need to take steps to stop the itching so that you can stop scratching. The best way to do this is to apply a wet compress that contains a couple of ice cubes. In many cases, a plain wet dressing made from water that contains a little salt or starch will relieve the itching.

How to Relieve Prickly Heat

An itching, burning rash around the chest, back, or waistline that occurs after prolonged sweating is usually prickly heat caused by obstruction of sweat ducts. A cool bath, or a warm tub bath containing a pound of boiled cornstarch, will usually relieve the itching. Taking 1,000 milligrams of Vitamin C daily during the summer may eliminate prickly heat entirely.

Common Sense Care for Intertrigo

Blondell M. threw away her bra when she became active in the women's liberation movement. "I'm not wearing a bra just to please men," she said. Unfortunately, Blondell's breasts sagged so much that the skin folded down to seal out air and seal in moisture. As a result, the skin under her breasts became raw and inflamed. I advised her to start wearing a bra again and to keep the inflamed skin dry and well ventilated. In just a few short weeks, the skin healed and the itching stopped.

Friction between moist skin surfaces anywhere on the body,

especially during the summer, will quickly erode the skin. The obvious remedy is to keep the skin surfaces dry and separated if possible. This can be done with powder, clothing, or a layer of cotton cloth. Dry and powder all the folds and crevices of your body after bathing. Expose your skin to sunlight occasionally. Remember, however, that perspiration will aggravate intertrigo. So don't sit in the sun and "sweat."

How to Relieve Housewife's Eczema

Many hard-working housewives suffer from housewife's eczema, which is characterized by itching, redness, and crusty formations around the hands and fingers. The cause of this condition is not usually known, but if the hands are protected from all the common household irritants the condition usually heals.

You can protect your hands by wearing rubber gloves over cotton gloves when performing wet chores, and by wearing cotton gloves when performing dry chores. Remove the gloves as soon as the chores are completed or when your hands begin to perspire. Moisture or perspiration inside the glove will aggravate the raw skin.

Itching can be relieved by immersing your hands in cold water that contains a little boiled cornstarch. If you feel that dry skin is the cause of your eczema, dip your hands into a pan of cold water that contains a tablespoonful of vegetable oil. In either case, let your hands dry by evaporation.

A Home-Care Program for Psoriasis

Dora K. was only 25 years of age when she began to notice little red bumps popping out on the skin of her hips and her abdomen. The red spots were soon replaced by large red patches that were covered with silvery scales. When one of the scales was peeled off, tiny pinpoints of blood could be seen. "It seems to be getting worse," she complained, "and my doctor says he doesn't know what's causing it."

Dora K. had psoriasis, a difficult-to-cure skin disease that will sometimes last a lifetime. Regular home care resulted in some immediate improvement in the appearance of her skin, and the glistening red patches slowly began to disappear. Follow these suggestions for a similar home-care program:

1. *Benefit from the healing powers of the sun.* Two or three times a week, expose your skin gradually to sunlight or ultraviolet rays. Sunlight, without perspiration, helps most skin diseases, particularly psoriasis. There are, however, a few skin diseases, such as lupus erythematosus, that are aggravated by the sun's rays. There are some people who develop fever blisters after over-exposure to ultraviolet rays from the sun or from a lamp.

2. *Enrich your diet and control your fat intake.* You can get the essential fatty acids you need by using a good cold-pressed vegetable oil on your salads. Take 50,000 units of Vitamin A daily for a few months, along with Vitamin B and lecithin for better fat metabolism. It might, in fact, be a good idea to increase your intake of all the natural food supplements that are rich in the basic vitamins and minerals.

Occasionally rub a little wheat germ oil over the diseased skin.

Cut down on animal fat, and eliminate processed foods containing saturated fat. Butter, lard, coconut oil, and hydrogenated vegetable oil, for example, are saturated fats.

Some doctors have suggested that all meats should be boiled for five minutes to eliminate taurine, a non-essential amino acid that may contribute to the development of psoriasis. Boiling, however, will wash the B vitamins out of the meat, making it even more necessary to take a Vitamin B supplement. Soybeans can replace meat occasionally, since they are low in taurine but rich in protein.

3. *Clean and bathe diseased skin daily.* Each day, bathe and remove all scales with a soft skin brush. If the use of a mild soap seems to aggravate the condition or cause itching, bathe in oatmeal water and use bran, oatmeal flakes, or a bag of oatmeal as an abrasive. Cold, wet dressings containing oatmeal water will often relieve itching. Shampoo your scalp at least three times weekly.

How to Handle Greasy-Scale Dermatitis

In seborrheic dermatitis, the affected skin, usually around the face and scalp or under the arms and between the thighs, is covered with red patches and greasy, yellowish scales. Frequent bathing will be necessary to keep the skin clean and dry. Concentrate on a high-protein diet that contains a minimum amount of fat and oil. Supplements containing Vitamin B and Vitamin C complex may aid recovery.

First Aid for Poison Ivy

If you're ever exposed to a vine that has three leaves on a red-flicked stem, you should rush home, wash your skin with a strong alkali soap, and then douse your body with rubbing alcohol. If you can do this within 30 minutes after the exposure, you may be able to avoid the itching rash and blisters that result from poison ivy.

If the blisters do appear, you should discontinue the use of soap. Cold baths and wet dressings will relieve discomfort. A boiled starch or oatmeal solution, or a paste made from baking soda and water, will relieve itching if applied directly to the skin.

The course of poison ivy can be shortened by taking the tops off the blisters. Wipe the skin clean with rubbing alcohol and then use a sterilized needle to open the blisters. Don't worry about spreading the infection. The fluid in the blisters is not contagious.

What to Do About White Skin Patches

Jerome A. was a healthy-looking man of 33, but he had suddenly started developing white patches on his hands and arms. He first noticed them after spending a long-awaited vacation at a lake resort. "There must be something terribly wrong," he said. "Do you think I might have leprosy or something like that?"

Jerome had a condition known as vitiligo, a harmless loss of pigmentation in the skin. It's not usually associated with disease, and the cause is not usually known. There have been reports, however, of people who have restored the pigmentation with natural foods, such as liver and brewer's yeast, that are rich in B vitamins.

The white patches become more evident when the skin is tanned by the sun. The reason for this, of course, is that the white patches do not contain enough pigment to respond to the sun's rays, while the surrounding skin tans normally. Some people stain the patches with diluted iodine or with the juice of green walnut hulls.

Miscellaneous Remedies for a Variety of Skin, Nail, and Hair Disorders

Sunburn

Soaking in a tub of cool water, or dousing your body with rubbing alcohol or witch hazel, will relieve the searing pain of a sunburn. Sponging the skin with vinegar *before* blisters develop might also help.

Blistered skin can be dabbed with olive oil or a mixture of mineral oil and menthol. Bathing in a tub of water containing oatmeal powder often proves to be soothing. A paste made from water and sodium bicarbonate is sometimes applied to badly burned skin. The pain of a simple burn is best relieved with plain cold water or an ice pack.

Note: If you use a lotion to prevent sunburn, select one that contains para-aminobenzoic acid.

Boils

Fold a cloth or piece of flannel and wring it out in a quart of hot water that contains two tablespoons of Epsom salts. Lay the cloth over the boil. Repeat the application when the cloth cools, or simply pour a little of the hot water on the cloth while it's laying over the boil. A hand or a foot may simply be immersed in the water.

The Epsom salts water will draw the pus to the surface so that it can drain. A yellow or white tip on a boil may be pricked with a sterilized needle. Squeezing a boil might create a more serious infection (a carbuncle) by forcing the infection deeper into the tissues. It may be all right to aid draining by pulling the skin down on each side of the boil to create a little pressure, but you should never pinch a boil.

Note: If you have boils and infections frequently, reduce the amount of sugar in your diet and be tested for diabetes.

Warts

A wart will sometimes disappear if it is kept covered with adhesive tape to shut out air and light and to prevent irritation. Soaking the wart in warm water might also help. Some doctors recommend rubbing a wart with castor oil three or four times a day.

Head lice

The eggs of head lice are usually attached to the base of the hairs near the scalp, and they are difficult or impossible to remove by washing. It may be necessary to clip the hair or soak the scalp with equal parts of olive oil and kerosene in order to get rid of the eggs. Hot vinegar will sometimes loosen the eggs so that they can be combed from the hair with a fine-toothed comb.

Remember that lice can be transmitted by personal contact. Be sure to avoid using hats, combs, wigs, hairbrushes, and other objects that have been used by someone who has head or body lice. Children who sit with the back of their head resting against the top of a theater seat sometimes pick up head lice.

Ticks

When a tick buries its head in your skin, it must not be removed forcefully. Pulling it off with your fingers, for example, may leave its head behind—buried deeply in your flesh. This could lead to the formation of a "skin knot" or an infection that might require medical care.

Touching a burning cigarette to a tick may force it to back out and drop from your skin. A drop of gasoline might also do the trick. Covering the insect with a glob of Vaseline petroleum jelly for 10 to 15 minutes might suffocate it so that it will release its grip. Whatever method you use, give the tick time to withdraw from your skin.

Unwanted hair

Women who want to remove unwanted body hair without shaving or using a chemical hair remover can use a wax depilatory.

A special wax purchased at cosmetic stores is heated and then painted over the skin and covered with a strip of cloth. When the wax hardens, the cloth and the wax are ripped off together, leaving the skin smooth and free of visible hair. The hair grows back in about three weeks, but in areas like the upper lip, where shaving would leave a stubble, wax depilation may do more for romance and femininity. Fine, black hair can sometimes be concealed by bleaching.

Baldness

Some men inherit male pattern baldness that is caused by the influence of male hormones. The only cure for this type of baldness is castration—*before* baldness occurs. No man would give up his manhood in order to keep his hair.

In some cases, baldness occurs simply because the scalp gets so tight that the flow of blood to the hair roots is restricted. This can be corrected by loosening the scalp with fingertip massage. Try to *stretch* the skin of your scalp by rolling it around and pinching it up with your fingertips. Don't wear hats that squeeze your head. Shampoo as often as necessary to remove excessive oil and dandruff. Dandruff doesn't cause baldness, but the caking of dirt, grease, and dead tissue cells on the scalp will certainly have a bad effect on the hair roots.

One nutritionist recommends inositol, a B vitamin, for baldness. She reports that in many cases bald spots were completely covered by a new growth of hair after supplementing the diet with inositol mixed into fortified milk. A teaspoonful of pure inositol was added to a quart of milk containing one teaspoonful of brewer's yeast powder, one-half cup of powdered milk, one tablespoonful of vegetable oil, one-half teaspoonful of magnesium oxide, one tablespoonful of lecithin granules, one raw egg, and one-half cup of frozen fruit juice concentrate. That is certainly a nutritious drink that should be of value to anyone, bald or not!

Dandruff

Wash or shampoo your scalp at least three times a week. And each time you wash, repeat the soaping and rinsing two or three times to remove the oil and dead skin that is caked on your scalp. If you must wash with hard water, rinsing your hair with water that contains a little vinegar will wash away the film that forms when soap and hard water are combined. The vinegar solution may then be washed away with fresh water. A little olive oil can be used to relieve dryness following a shampoo.

Brush your hair and scalp for two or three minutes each night to remove dirt and scales. Use a soft brush so that you won't break the hairs or irritate your scalp. I recommend that you do not use a brush that has nylon bristles.

Brittle nails

Twice each day, take two teaspoons of gelatin that have been dissolved in a glass of warm water. Although gelatin is not a complete protein, studies have shown that gelatin *does* strengthen nails in some mysterious way.

Brittle nails can also result from an iodine deficiency. Seafood supplies complete protein as well as the iodine you need for healthy nails.

Fingernails sometimes become dry and cracked after prolonged use of nail-polish remover, detergents, and other artificial products. Soaking the nails in water and then coating them with oil will help restore their moisture content.

Weeping, inflamed skin

Cool, wet applications will usually relieve the moist-type skin inflammation that occurs in such conditions as eczema. Wring out cloths in water that contains one teaspoonful of salt for each pint of water.

Prolonged cool baths, with or without cornstarch or oatmeal, are soothing to inflamed skin. Mixing a coal tar solution into the bath water may be helpful.

Bed sores

If you must be confined to bed for a long period of time, there's plenty that you can do to keep bed sores from developing. Get a foam-rubber mattress—or pad your mattress with a layer of foam rubber—and then use a variety of sleeping postures. Make sure that there are no wrinkles in the sheet. When you're lying on your back, a pillow under both of your knees will relieve pressure on the back of your heels. Dry your skin thoroughly after each bath. An alcohol massage each day will harden your skin and stimulate healing circulation. If a sore does develop, keep bed pressures off the sore and supplement your diet with high-protein powder, Vitamin A, and Vitamin C.

Impetigo

If blisters form anywhere on your body for no apparent reason (especially around your face, scalp, hands, and arms) and then break to form a thick yellowish crust, you may have impetigo. This is a highly contagious infection that can be transmitted by direct contact.

Keep your body as clean as possible, and change towels, linen, and clothing each day. Remove the crusts on the sores by scrubbing with soap and water or by rubbing them with cotton soaked in alcohol. After bathing, or after cleaning an individual sore, sponge the skin with alcohol.

Eat vitamin-rich natural foods and supplement your diet with the essential vitamins.

Avoid contact with other members of your family, sleep alone, and use separate washcloths and towels.

Insect stings

When you are bitten by a bee, a spider, or some other insect, an ice bag or a cold compress will relieve pain and swelling. Wring out a towel in ice water that contains a couple tablespoons of bicarbonate of soda. If you like, you may wrap a couple of ice cubes in the towel.

Remove stingers by scraping the skin with a dull knife. Gripping the end of a stinger with your fingers may only inject the remaining poison from the stinger into your body.

Summary

1. When the use of mildly alkaline soap seems to aggravate dry skin, go easy on soap and rub your skin with oil after each bath.
2. Oily skin should be washed frequently with alkaline soap.
3. Sunlight, frequent washing, and a good diet are all helpful in overcoming acne.
4. Itching skin can be relieved by bathing in water containing boiled cornstarch, cooked oatmeal, or sodium bicarbonate.
5. Housewife's eczema will usually clear up if the hands are protected from contact with common household irritants.
6. Psoriasis will respond to sunlight, coal tar, and dietary measures if the silvery scales are removed by regular bathing.
7. If white patches on the skin do not respond to an enriched diet, they are sometimes stained for cosmetic reasons.
8. The pain of sunburn can be relieved by soaking in a tub of cool water or by sponging the body with alcohol, witch hazel, or vinegar.
9. Hot compresses soaked with Epsom salts water will speed the drainage of boils.
10. The miscellaneous home remedies at the end of this chapter cover a variety of ailments from bed sores to baldness.

12

How to Relieve Fatigue and Rejuvenate Your Body with Massage and Naturomatic Tonics

"Chronic fatigue" is one of the most common complaints we hear these days, both inside and outside doctors' offices. There are many causes of fatigue, some of which can be handled better at home than in a doctor's office. There are numerous natural tonics that you and your family can use to relieve fatigue and restore energy. You'll learn about some of these tonics in this chapter, and what you learn will prove to be of great value to you in meeting the stress and routine of everyday living.

How to Eliminate Fatigue Caused by Hypoglycemia (Low Blood Sugar)

Most people think that when they need a little energy all they have to do is eat or drink something containing sugar. It's true that sugar will sometimes relieve fatigue by raising the blood sugar level, but it can also contribute to the development of a more serious form of fatigue.

Hypoglycemia is a fatiguing blood-sugar deficiency that is sometimes triggered by an excessive amount of refined sugar or white flour in the diet. The glucose supplied by these refined carbohydrates is absorbed into the system so rapidly that there is a sudden and abnormal rise in blood sugar. This forces the pancreas to release so much insulin that there is a drastic *drop* in blood sugar about four hours after eating. Since low blood sugar or hypoglycemia is accompanied by weakness, fatigue, headache, trembling, hunger, and other symptoms of sugar starvation, the victim usually craves something sweet. If he eats something containing white sugar or white flour, his blood sugar will shoot up again for awhile and then fall again a few hours later. This results in a see-sawing blood sugar and a constant craving for sweets, and it leads to overweight, heart disease, diabetes, arthritis, allergies, and other diseases. Following are guidelines for coping with this type of fatigue.

Quit eating refined carbohydrates!

Whether you suffer from hypoglycemia or not, you should quit eating foods that contain refined sugar or white flour. This step alone will usually eliminate the midmorning and midafternoon fatigue that results from a fall in blood sugar.

Eat six times a day

If you continue to experience fatigue and other symptoms of low blood sugar in spite of eating meals made up of fresh, natural foods, you may have to eat six small meals each day rather than three large meals. Or you may have to snack between meals as a supplement only to your "regular" meal schedule.

How to control your blood sugar
with natural food snacks

Fresh fruits or unsweetened fruit juices contain fructose, a form of fruit sugar that can raise your blood sugar without over-stimulating your pancreas.

Protein foods supply long-lasting energy without flooding the blood with sugar. Such foods as baked chicken, cottage cheese, skim milk, natural peanut butter with crackers, seeds, nuts, or toasted soybeans, for example, can be used to supply energy between meals.

If you must have sweets, eat dried fruits, but eat them sparingly. A little honey stirred into a glass of orange juice will supply quick energy for athletes and other persons who have exhausted their blood sugar in physical activity.

How to relieve mental and muscular fatigue with food

The brain and the muscles need glucose to function. When blood sugar falls because of the reaction of a sensitive pancreas to sugar-rich foods, it may fall so low that both the brain and the muscles become fatigued. Marvin C., for example, complained of "rubbery legs" and an inability to concentrate. "I get so tired and shaky," he said, "that I can hardly complete my sales route each day. And my brain gets so foggy that I cannot make an effective sales pitch."

A check of Marvin's eating habits revealed that his diet was heavy in refined sugar and starches. When he switched to a high-protein diet with plenty of fresh fruits and vegetables, his fatigue vanished and his sales improved. "I snack on fresh fruit and toasted soybeans between meals," he reported. "I feel like a new man, and I no longer feel the need to stuff myself at mealtime."

Note: Don't drink coffee, tea, or cola drinks between meals for a "lift," even if they do not contain sugar. These beverages contain caffeine and other stimulants that may *lower* blood sugar by triggering a chain reaction that begins with stimulation of the adrenal glands.

Lying on a *slant board* with your feet at the high end of the board will relieve mental fatigue by bathing your brain with a fresh supply of blood, oxygen, and glucose.

How to Use Diet to Relieve Fatigue Caused by Diabetes

When the pancreas is constantly abused or overworked from excessive use of sugar, it eventually becomes exhausted and fails to produce enough insulin to cope with large amounts of sugar. Then, what began as low blood sugar from an overproduction of insulin becomes diabetes or *high* blood sugar from a deficiency of insulin. In either case, you'll have to *avoid sugar and refined carbohydrates* and go easy on natural starches in order to keep your blood sugar under control. With the average American consuming about 150 pounds of sugar annually, it's no wonder hypoglycemia and diabetes are so common. Hypoglycemia is rarely detected and treated by physicians, but diabetes is often detected in routine medical examinations.

The medicinal value
of green vegetables

Green leafy vegetables contain myrtillin, which helps lower blood sugar. Blueberry and huckleberry leaves are especially rich in myrtillin, and may be used to make a beverage for use with meals. You may gather your own leaves for steeping in hot water, or you may purchase them in dry tea form in health food stores.

Balancing diet and insulin

There are some diabetics who are so deficient in insulin that they must have insulin injections to utilize blood sugar for energy. These people should be under the care of a physician so that blood sugar measurements can be used to determine the amount of insulin they need. It's still important, however, that they eat fresh, natural foods and stay away from refined sugars and starches. The less sugar there is in the blood, the smaller the doses of insulin. Some "diabetics" are even able to quit taking insulin when they change their eating habits.

Diabetes that begins in middle age can be controlled by diet alone in most cases. This means that in addition to restricting sugar and starches, a special effort should be made to eat such basic natural foods as lean meat, fish, poultry, eggs, fruits, vegetables, milk products, and whole grain cereals. Such foods won't flood your blood with sugar, and they'll supply the vitamins and minerals your body needs to improve the function of your pancreas. An occasional blood sugar examination by your doctor will help you evaluate your eating habits. Frequent urination, excessive thirst, itching, hunger, weakness, and weight loss may mean that diabetes is getting out of control.

Note: When diabetes is advanced, your body will begin to eliminate sugar in your urine. You can test for urine sugar right in your own home with a "Clinitest kit" or similar kit that can be purchased in any drug store without a prescription. Many diabetics use this test to measure the effects of the foods they eat.

How to boost a diabetic diet's efficiency with food supplements

Natural food supplements can be used to overcome nutritional deficiencies and to boost the healing powers of the body. The B vitamins, for example, aid carbohydrate metabolism and decrease the need for insulin. Brewer's yeast and wheat germ are rich in B vitamins. Since the liver of a diabetic may have trouble converting vegetable carotene to Vitamin A, fish liver oil will be helpful in maintaining Vitamin A stores. Water-soluble Vitamins B and C, lost because of excessive thirst and frequent urination, may have to be replaced with vitamin supplements.

Substituting unsaturated vegetable fat for animal fat in the diet helps to regulate blood sugar as well as prevent the development of diabetic arteriosclerosis. Nuts, avocados, sunflower seeds, vegetable oil, and fish supply essential fatty acids as well as important vitamins and minerals.

In diabetes, as in any other disease, it's important to make sure that the body is fortified with all the food elements it needs to overcome deficiencies and to function with a handicap.

How to Relieve Fatigue Caused by Iron-Deficient Blood

Anemia is another common cause of fatigue that can be corrected with dietary measures. When the blood cells are deficient in iron, they cannot transport enough oxygen to the tissue cells of your body. This can result in shortness of breath, headache, numbness, neuritis, faintness, dizziness, and other symptoms as well as chronic fatigue.

Mary Ann B. had complained of fatigue and weakness for a number of years. "My husband accuses me of being lazy," she said, "and my doctor says I'm having trouble with my nerves. I'm just tired all the time, and sometimes my hands and feet tingle." I asked her if she had ever been checked for anemia. "I was anemic several years ago," she replied, "but it was corrected with iron pills." Mary Ann didn't know it, but she was losing more iron in her heavy menstrual flow each month than she was getting in her diet. When she added a little extra iron to her diet, her fatigue disappeared and her energy zoomed. "I feel so much better now than I did a month ago," she reported, "that I'm looking for a job. Now it's my husband who is always complaining about being 'too tired'."

Foods are your best sources of iron

Liver, muscle meats, egg yolk, dark molasses, green leafy vegetables, and dried fruits are good sources of iron. Wheat germ and brewer's yeast are rich in iron, and may be added to foods or used as supplements. Parsley is so rich in iron that it should be a part of every fresh salad that is served in your home.

Except in cases of blood loss, as in injury or heavy menstruation, you can get all the iron you need from natural foods. Your body conserves iron by using the same iron over and over to build new blood cells from old, worn-out blood cells. You should, however, try to make sure that your diet contains at least 15 milligrams of iron each day. If you get your iron from natural foods rather than from "iron enriched" refined foods, it's not likely that you'll take in a harmful or excessive amount of iron.

A two-ounce piece of pork liver contains about 15 milligrams of iron; one-half cup of wheat germ, about 6.4 milligrams; one tablespoonful of brewer's yeast, about 2 milligrams; five dried apricots, 4.6 milligrams; and one-half cup of parsley, 9.6 milligrams.

A variety of foods is essential in combating anemia

It's important to remember that many other vitamins and minerals, such as Vitamin B and copper, are necessary for the absorption and utilization of iron. So it will be necessary to eat a variety of natural foods to correct iron-deficiency anemia. A vegetarian, for example, who does not include milk, cheese, fish, or eggs in his diet may develop symptoms of pernicious anemia from a Vitamin B_{12} deficiency. (Vitamin B_{12} is found almost exclusively in foods of animal origin.)

Stomach acid is needed for absorption of iron and Vitamin B $_{12}$

Persons who have a hydrochloric acid deficiency in their stomach may develop pernicious anemia because of their ability to absorb iron and Vitamin B_{12}. Glutamic hydrochloric acid tablets, or a half-teaspoon of dilute hydrochloric acid mixed in half a glass of water (or buttermilk) and sipped through a straw (to protect the teeth) during meals will aid absorption of iron. In severe cases of pernicious anemia, however, a physician may have to inject the body with liver extract or Vitamin B_{12}. Supplements (brewer's yeast, wheat germ, desiccated liver) containing B vitamins will help the body produce its own hydrochloric acid.

Breathing Carbon Monoxide Can Cause Fatigue

If you are a heavy smoker, or if you breathe air containing the exhaust fumes of heaters and engines, you might suffer from fatigue caused by carbon monoxide poisoning. Your red blood cells will quickly absorb the carbon monoxide that is breathed into your lungs. This reduces the number of blood cells that are available for carrying oxygen and eliminating wastes.

Take advantage of every opportunity to get to breathe fresh, clean air. Breathe deeply into your abdomen and then high up into your chest to assure ventilation of all the lobes of your lungs. Don't take more than two or three deep breaths at one time, however, so that you won't experience dizziness and other symptoms of hyperventilation.

How to Remove Poisons and Wake Up Your Body with Stimulating Massage

Most people think of massage as a method of relieving tension and relaxing muscles. It can also be used to relieve fatigue and wake up your body—depending upon how the massage is given. When a massage is gentle, your muscles respond by relaxing. But when massage is vigorous, the stimulation of nerves and the movement of a large volume of blood serves as a tonic that sharpens your senses and restores your energy.

Doug C. is a hard-driving businessman who frequently uses massage to rejuvenate his aching body. "When I'm bone tired at the end of the day and I have to make a sales presentation at night, I get a vigorous massage and I'm raring to go. In fact, I don't believe that I could get by without an occasional massage."

If you aren't able to get the services of a professional masseur, you can teach any member of your family how to give a simple massage.

How to massage your muscles at home

When you are in a hurry, a massage from the waist up is all that's necessary for a tonic effect.

Quick, overlapping strokes that are applied with fairly heavy pressure will prove to be stimulating to the muscles. A small amount of lubricant on the skin will reduce friction and make the massage more comfortable. Baby oil, vegetable oil, mineral oil, cocoa butter, or a little oil mixed with alcohol will do.

Lie on your back and instruct the person giving the massage to follow this procedure:

> *Arms:* Begin at the wrist of one arm. Work up the arm by kneading and squeezing with your thumb and fingers on each side of the arm. Use short, overlapping strokes until the entire arm is covered. Then grasp the wrist with one hand and use the opposite hand to massage the arm with one long stroke from the wrist to the shoulder. Repeat the stroke three or four times, making sure that you cover all sides of the arm.
>
> Follow the same procedure for the opposite arm.
>
> *Abdomen:* Massage the abdomen by placing both hands flat on the abdomen and moving them in a circular motion. This can be done best without a lubricant so that your hands won't slip. Just keep the palms of your hands in firm contact with the skin so that the flesh moves with your hands. Move your left hand in a clockwise motion and your right hand in a counterclockwise motion.

Chest: The technique used to massage the abdomen can be used to massage the muscles of a man's chest. A woman's breasts, however, should not be massaged. Instead, she may contract the muscles lying underneath her breasts by pressing her hands together in front of her chest several times.

Neck: Place the fingers of both hands behind the ears on each side of the neck and stroke downward and forward over the neck toward the breast bone. Repeat several times.

The neck massage is taken in a face-up position, but the rest of the massage is taken in a face-down position.

Back: Place both hands on the muscles on each side of the spinal column and rub from bottom to top in short, overlapping strokes. Repeat three or four times, and then stroke from bottom to top in one continuous movement.

For the muscles in the shoulder-blade area, place one hand on each side of the back just beneath the shoulder blades. Then, with the hands in firm contact with the skin, move the left hand in a circular clockwise motion and the right hand in a circular counterclockwise motion. Roll the muscles in this fashion for several seconds.

Neck and shoulders: Place one hand on each side of the neck and stroke downward toward the tip of the shoulder. Repeat three or four times. Finish with repeated, rapid squeezing of the thick muscles that lie midway between the neck and the shoulder on each side.

How to stimulate the spinal nerves

A little vibration or jarring of the spinal column at the conclusion of a vigorous massage will stimulate the spinal nerves for a maximum amount of get-up-and-go. If you don't have a vibrator that you can run up and down the spine, you can use this technique: Straddle the spinal column with the first two fingers of one hand and then pound the fingers with the bottom of a closed fist. The vibration will be transmitted from the fingers to the spine, and the fingers will protect the bony areas of the spine from direct blows. Start in the upper back area and work down to the pelvic portion of the spine. Pound just hard enough to get a comfortable stimulation. Stop if any pain or discomfort results.

If you can stand the shock, rubbing an ice cube up and down your spine will really wake you up.

After the massage has been completed, the oil on the skin can be removed with rubbing alcohol, which in itself will have tonic effects.

How to Relieve Fatigue with Water Tonics

Plain cold water applied to your body is one of the quickest and most potent tonics you can use at home for stimulating nerves and overcoming fatigue. Bathing or sponging with cold water, for example, will increase your working ability about 30 percent—and it will boost your mental capacity as well. Too long an exposure to cold water, however, can be overstimulating and fatiguing. So for tonic purposes, treatment with cold water should be brief—rarely longer than a minute or two. And the older you are, the shorter the exposure should be.

The cold shower tonic

A simple cold-water shower that is preceded by a warm shower gradually turned to a comfortably cold temperature is the simplest way to stimulate the body with water. Persons who have a good circulatory reaction can benefit from a plunge into a pool of cold water immediately following a hot shower.

Water colder than 60 degrees Fahrenheit will be too cold for the average person. If you suffer a chill, or if your skin turns blue rather than pink following immersion in cold water, you'll know that the water is too cold for you, regardless of its temperature. If your nerves and your circulation react the way they should, you'll be bursting with energy after a cold shower or a cold-water plunge.

The cold mitten friction

Rubbing your body with towel mittens that have been dipped in ice water is a convenient and effective way to get all the benefits of a cold-water tonic. First take a brief hot shower so that circulatory reaction will protect you against chilling. Then sit down in the tub and place a pan of cold water (50 to 60 degrees F.) between your legs. Dip your mitten-covered hands into the water and begin rubbing your body—one part at a time—until you have covered your entire body. Rub briskly until the skin glows with a pleasant pink color.

You can increase the tonic effects of a mitten rub by frequently dipping the mittens into the cold water—depending upon how well you tolerate the cold.

Dry your body vigorously with a coarse Turkish towel.

How to Use a Wet Sheet Rub for Instant Vigor

The wet-sheet rub is a vigorous tonic that will quickly pep you up. You'll need a helper, however, to apply the sheet and to rub your body.

Gather these materials before you begin: two sheets, a large pan containing enough hot water (105 degrees F.) to cover your feet, a pail of cold water (60 to 70 degrees F.), two long strips of towel, a pail of ice water, and a Turkish towel.

A wet sheet technique for home use

Strip down until nude (or to your shorts) and stand in the pan of hot water.

Wring out two strips of towel in the ice water and then wrap one strip around your head and the other around your neck.

Have your helper wring out a sheet lightly in the cold water and then wrap it around your body in the following manner: Hold up both of your arms. Place the upper corner of one side of the sheet under your left arm and then lower that arm to hold the sheet in place. Wrap the sheet around your chest and back and then lower your right arm. The sheet is then wrapped over your arms, chest, and shoulders and around your neck so that it can be tucked under the edge of the sheet behind your neck.

Instruct your helper to rub and slap the sheet vigorously over your entire body until the sheet becomes warm. The trick is to rub the sheet without making it slide over your skin. Your helper should work fast so that your body won't have a chance to get chilled.

Dry your body by replacing the wet sheet with a warm, dry

sheet for a dry-sheet rub. Finish by rubbing your body vigorously with a Turkish towel.

A man and his wife who help each other with a wet-sheet rub told me that the treatment was a twice-weekly ritual in their home. "When we need a little extra vigor," they said, "we can always depend upon that cold sheet to really pep us up. Until we started using the wet-sheet rub, we just didn't have enough energy to do all the things we wanted to do. Now we have as much energy as high-school newlyweds!"

How to Relieve Sexual Fatigue with a Sitz Bath

When I asked one of my patients for the secret of his father's success as a newlywed at the age of 70, he replied: "My father sits in a sitz bath every day."

There actually is some evidence to indicate that a cold sitz bath will stimulate sexual powers or relieve sexual fatigue. All you have to do is fill your tub with just enough cold water to cover your knuckles when you touch the bottom of the tub with the tip of your middle finger. You can put a few ice cubes into the water for a more stimulating effect. Sit in the water with your knees bent so that only your buttocks and your feet are submerged. Remain in the water for about 15 minutes.

One famous physician has suggested that a "sexually tired" man might be able to rejuvenate himself by dipping his testicles into a glass of ice water!

Note: Pumpkin seeds and the sarsaparilla root contain a substance resembling the male hormone, testosterone. Some doctors believe that the hormones in pumpkin seeds improve the health of the prostate gland.

A "Tiger's Milk" Cocktail for Quick Energy

For a highly-nourishing quick-energy drink, mix one quart of milk with one-half cup of dried milk, one-half cup of brewer's yeast powder, and a small can of frozen, concentrated orange juice. Mix in a blender and keep in a refrigerator for use as a pick-me-up beverage. If you like, you may add a raw egg yolk for additional enrichment. Any frozen fruit juice concentrate may be used for flavor. Or you may use ripe bananas or peaches.

Tiger's milk is rich in B vitamins, protein, iron, Vitamin C, and other elements you need for quick energy and good health. Many people use Tiger's milk as a breakfast drink. One of my patients, a 45-year-old social worker who spends long hours each day working with problem families, maintains that Tiger's milk gives her the "push" she needs to keep up with her grueling schedule. "I have more than enough energy to do my work each day and then go home and take care of my family. I feel sure that it's the brewer's yeast that gives me all that energy."

It's well known that Vitamin B_1 (thiamine) acts as a tonic by converting glucose into energy and by disposing of pyruvic acid and lactic acid waste products. *Brewer's yeast is rich in B vitamins,* including thiamine. If you prefer to take vitamin pills, you should take *Vitamin B complex,* since *all* the B vitamins work together. Taking only one B vitamin may result in a deficiency in some of the other B vitamins.

Summary

1. Fatigue, weakness, trembling, and other symptoms of hypoglycemia can usually be relieved by avoiding white sugar and white-flour products.
2. Between-meal snacks of fresh fruit and protein-rich foods will maintain energy levels without overstimulating your pancreas.
3. Diabetes that occurs after middle age can usually be controlled with a diet consisting solely of natural foods.
4. Except in cases of blood loss, the iron supplied by meat, green leafy vegetables, dried fruits, and other natural foods will be adequate for correcting iron-deficiency anemia.
5. Persons suffering from pernicious anemia may have to supplement their diet with hydrochloric acid tablets and Vitamin B_{12}.
6. Breathing air containing carbon monoxide causes fatigue and other symptoms by preventing the red blood cells from absorbing oxygen.
7. A vigorous massage will wake up your body by stimulating nerves and increasing the flow of blood.

8. A cold shower, a cold-mitten friction, or a wet-sheet rub will give you quick energy and new vigor.
9. A cold sitz bath will do wonders in overcoming sexual fatigue.
10. A Tiger's milk cocktail is a highly nourishing pick-me-up beverage that will build health as well as supply energy.

13

How to Reverse the Causes
of Premature Aging and
Remain Younger Longer
with Naturomatic Healing

Few people think of old age as a disease. The truth is, however, that old age as we know it *is* a disease. All the diseases and aches and pains that now kill or cripple "old" people are not a normal part of the aging process. *A person who is truly healthy should grow old without suffering from the process of aging,* and he should live *longer* than a hundred years. Biologists say that the human body should last at least 125 years or even 150 years.

Unfortunately, few people actually die of old age. Just about everyone dies prematurely from heart trouble, cancer, hardened arteries, and other diseases that are caused by bad living habits. Dr. Hans Selye, the famous physician who proved that stress was a major cause of disease, wrote in his book, *The Stress of Life* (McGraw-Hill), that in all the autopsies he has performed he has never seen a case of death caused by old age. "In fact," he wrote, "I do not think anyone has died of old age yet . . . . To die of old age would mean that all the organs of the body would be worn out proportionately, merely by having been used too long. This is never the case. We invariably die because one vital part has worn out too early in proportion to the rest of the body."

Anything that promotes good health will combat the aging

202

process. There are, however, some special measures that you should use *daily* to make sure that your tissue cells receive all the elements they need to resist disease and aging. *Good nutrition alone is a potent remedy for premature aging,* and it will reverse the course of many common diseases that cause an organ to fail prematurely.

Improved circulation will aid transportation of nutrients to tissue cells and improve "cell respiration." Natural tonics and remedies for weakness, fatigue, sluggishness, insomnia, and other symptoms pointing to premature aging will improve your health and lengthen your life.

Remember that each year 98 percent of the atoms in your body are replaced by new atoms from food, air, and water. This means that you must make sure that your body is well nourished and properly cared for day after day and year after year. Even if you aren't now "old" or sick, you should begin *now* to reverse the processes that cause premature aging and death.

Nutritional Remedies for Aging, Sagging Tissue

Claudia B. was only 34 years of age when she began to notice that her flesh was sagging. "My husband says my skin looks like crepe paper," she complained. "And I'm beginning to look older than my mother." I told Claudia how important good nutrition was for building and maintaining firm and healthy tissue. For the first time in her life she started eating fresh, natural foods. The changes in her physical appearance were remarkable. In a few short months, she looked years younger—and she *was* younger. What brought about this change? The vitamins, minerals, and enzymes in *living* food.

How to Use Vitamin C to Strengthen Tissue Cells

It's now well known that Vitamin C strengthens tissue cells by supplying them with a special "cement" that holds them together. It also strengthens the collagen or connective tissue that keeps your flesh from sagging. Since your body doesn't store Vitamin C, you need a new supply each day—and the more you can get from natural foods the better.

Laboratory experiments with animals have revealed that the younger the animal the greater the concentration of Vitamin C in its tissues. And according to the U.S. Department of Agriculture, "The higher concentration of Vitamin C in young tissues than in old and the high concentration in actively multiplying cells and tissue indicate that Vitamin C must be present where tissue is formed or regenerated." You should make sure that your body has all the Vitamin C it needs to keep your tissues strong and healthy, which will prevent disease as well as delay the aging process. Vitamin C is, in fact, so effective in building youthful health that it is sometimes called "the beauty and youth vitamin."

Natural food sources of Vitamin C

All types of fresh fruits and vegetables contain Vitamin C. Citrus fruits, tomatoes, cabbage, melons, green peppers, strawberries, and parsley, for example, are good sources of Vitamin C. Since Vitamin C can be destroyed by heat and washed out by water, you cannot depend upon cooked vegetables for all the Vitamin C you need to overcome the effects of premature aging. You must eat plenty of whole, fresh fruit. Whenever possible, such vegetables as tomatoes, cucumbers, celery, and cabbage should also be eaten raw. Fresh fruit and vegetable juices, or pureed fruits and vegetables, are helpful when dental problems do not permit adequate chewing.

Sprouted grains, seeds, or beans are tremendously rich in Vitamin C. They contain the germ of life. Mix the raw sprouts in with regular salads. Any health food store can get you started in growing your own sprouts. It's a simple process that takes only a few days. Basically, all you have to do is wrap a few beans in a towel and then pour warm water over them several times a day until they sprout.

Natural Vitamin C supplements made from rose hips, acerola cherries, and green peppers will provide you with potent Vitamin C insurance. If you do take a Vitamin C supplement, you should take about 1,000 milligrams each day. It's important to take a *natural* supplement so you'll get the enzymes, bioflavonoids and other factors that will aid your body in using Vitamin C.

How to Get the "Rust" Out of Your Body with Vitamin E

Every tissue cell in your body needs oxygen to keep it alive. Without adequate Vitamin E, however, oxygen tends to oxidize or destroy essential fatty acids in the tissues, forming a peroxide substance that damages tissues and blood cells and results in premature aging. Like a piece of iron at the seashore, body tissues age or "rust" rapidly in the presence of oxygen when there is a deficiency in Vitamin E. (Vitamin C also protects the tissues from oxidation.)

Even the collagen or connective tissue that holds tissue cells together needs Vitamin E (and Vitamin C) to keep it flexible and healthy, giving it the elasticity of youth. And you need Vitamin E to protect Vitamin A, which you need for tight, youthful skin. You already know from reading Chapter 1 how important Vitamin E is in keeping the arteries and veins from becoming hard or clogged. With enough Vitamin E in your diet, you may be able to *reverse* some of the aging ailments that are already beginning to plague your body.

Natural food sources of Vitamin E

All types of fresh, natural foods, such as whole grains, wheat germ, seeds, nuts, leafy vegetables, fertile eggs, and meat contain some Vitamin E. Cold-pressed wheat germ oil is probably the best and the richest natural source of this important vitamin. Mix a tablespoonful or two in a raw vegetable salad each day—or take a natural Vitamin E supplement. See Chapter 14 for more information on Vitamin E.

How to Improve Cell Function with Calcium

When the body is deficient in calcium, the bones become brittle, nerves cannot function normally, contraction of the heart muscle is disturbed, and the tissue cells are unable to exchange wastes for nutrients. It's now well known that calcium deficiency causes premature aging—and surveys by the U.S. Department of Agriculture have revealed that Americans are often deficient in calcium! So if you show signs of premature aging, you'll want to increase your intake of calcium. It's important to remember, however, that you must also have Vitamin D, phosphorus, magnesium, and other vitamins and minerals to absorb and utilize calcium. Taking only calcium might even induce a deficiency in magnesium or some other companion mineral. This is one reason why you should eat a wide variety of natural foods, no matter what type of food supplement you take.

Many people take bone meal for calcium, since it contains all the minerals your body needs to build bone. Unfortunately, many "old" people are deficient in the stomach acid they need to absorb calcium. This means that they must take hydrochloric acid supplements with their meals, otherwise a vicious cycle of aging and calcium deficiency accelerates the aging process and contributes to the development of disease. (Squeezing lemon juice over foods will aid digestion and absorption of calcium.)

Natural food sources of calcium

Milk and milk products, green leafy vegetables, almonds, oysters, dried beans, and dark molasses are good sources of calcium.

Many people who have "calcium deposits" around painful joints feel that they should eliminate milk and other calcium rich foods in their diet. Most of the time, however, such calcium deposits have nothing to do with the amount of calcium in the diet. Even when the diet is deficient in calcium, the body will draw calcium from the bones to use in building formations around damaged joints. So in order to protect your bones, it's best to make sure that your diet contains adequate calcium, even if you do have "calcium spurs."

How to Prolong Your Life with Vitamin A

Dr. Henry Sherman of Columbia University once wrote that man could add *ten years* to his prime of life by eating four times the amount of Vitamin A recommended for the average person. This doesn't mean, however, that the more Vitamin A you get, the better. Vitamin A is a fat-soluble vitamin that can be stored in the body. You need all the Vitamin A you can get from natural foods, but too much from artificial sources can have toxic effects. So if you take a Vitamin A supplement, you should probably not take more than 25,000 units daily—certainly not more than 50,000 units. (The minimum daily requirement is 5,000 units.)

Natural food sources of Vitamin A

Vitamin A is found only in foods of animal origin, such as liver, butter, egg yolk, cheese, and whole milk. Two ounces of cooked beef liver supply more than 30,000 units of Vitamin A.

The carotene in yellow and green vegetables and yellow fruits can be converted into Vitamin A in the body. Some nutritionists say that the average adult who has a good diet gets about two-thirds of his daily Vitamin A requirement from carotene. If you're on a low-fat diet and you must restrict your intake of animal fat, you should probably add a little fish liver oil to your diet.

How to Get the Vitamin D You Need from Natural Sources

Vitamin D is also a fat-soluble vitamin that can be stored in the body. Like Vitamin A, it can have toxic effects when excessive amounts are taken in artificial form. Too much Vitamin D, for example, causes a build-up of calcium in the blood, which can damage joints, kidneys, blood vessels, and other structures. So you should make an effort to get the Vitamin D you need from sunlight, salt-water fish, egg yolk, liver, and enriched milk. Sunlight in the summer and cod liver oil in the winter should give you all the Vitamin D you need. (The minimum daily requirement is 400 units. More than 4,000 units daily is considered excessive for adults.)

A deficiency in Vitamin D can lead to soft bones, loose teeth, and other symptoms of premature aging.

How to Perk Up Your Nervous System with Vitamin B

Vitamin B is a water-soluble vitamin that's frequently washed out of foods in cooking, so the more of this vitamin you can get, the better. A deficiency can contribute to premature aging by weakening your nervous system and disturbing your metabolism. There are several B vitamins, and you need them all. This is why you should ask for "Vitamin B complex" when you buy a Vitamin B supplement.

Your body must have B vitamins to metabolize carbohydrate. This means that excessive use of refined carbohydrates, which do not contain B vitamins, will actually rob your body of vitamins. So always try to get your carbohydrate from vitamin-rich *natural* foods. You'll be rewarded with better health and a longer life.

Natural food sources of Vitamin B

Brewer's yeast is rich in B vitamins, and may be taken in tablet form or added to foods and beverages as a powder. Wheat germ, a delicious natural cereal, is also rich in B vitamins. Remember, however, that you must eat foods of animal origin for the Vitamin B_{12} you need to avoid the development of pernicious anemia.

Meat, liver, whole grain products, brown rice, sprouted grains, milk, eggs, cheese, fruits and vegetables contain some or all of the B vitamins. Desiccated liver is a good source of B vitamins, including Vitamin B_{12}, for persons who want all the benefits of liver without actually eating liver.

How to Strengthen Aging Tissues with Protein

The framework of every cell in your body is made of protein, and your muscles, nails, and hair are formed almost entirely from protein. Without adequate protein, your body shrinks, your ankles swell, your muscles become weak, your nails become brittle, and your hair falls out. Obviously, a protein deficiency can result in premature aging.

If you eat a variety of natural foods that include meat, fish, poultry, milk, eggs, or cheese, you won't ever be deficient in protein, and your body will be strong and well constructed. The average person needs about 70 grams of protein each day to maintain his tissues. This means that you must have a good serving of protein at each meal. And if you are to get the additional protein you need to be exceptionally strong, you should include such foods as soybeans, nuts, peas and beans, whole grains, and wheat germ. Sunflower seeds make a good between-meal protein snack.

Just to give you some idea of the protein content of the foods you eat, here is an analysis of some of the more popular foods: One cup of skim milk contains about nine grams of protein; one cup of cottage cheese, 38 grams of protein; one egg, 6 grams of protein; three ounces of beef or poultry, 24 grams of protein; three ounces of canned tuna, 25 grams of protein; one cup of beans, 15 grams of protein; one cup of roasted, shelled peanut halves, 39 grams of protein.

Obviously, you can get all the protein you need from the foods you eat. If you don't eat meat, you should at least eat such animal products as milk, eggs, and cheese. Some strict vegetarians who are trained in nutrition can combine a large number of different vegetables to form enough complete protein to meet their needs, but the average person cannot depend upon vegetables for his protein. If you don't think that you're getting enough protein from foods of animal origin, you should supplement your diet with a high-protein powder, which is very often made from soybeans.

Carbohydrates and Fats Also Combat the Aging Process

Plenty of fresh fruits, vegetables, and whole grain cereals will supply the carbohydrate you need for energy. There should be some carbohydrate in every meal, otherwise the body will be forced to burn fat for energy. And when fat is burned in the absence of carbohydrate, the fat is not completely oxidized, leaving an acid residue that has toxic effects. So don't ever try to lose weight by starving it off. You need some carbohydrate, even if you are on a reducing diet. Besides, when there is no carbo-hydrate in the diet, your body may also burn protein for energy—and you need all the protein you can get to combat the aging process.

In addition to supplying energy, aiding the oxidation of fat, and protecting protein, natural carbohydrates favor the growth of the intestinal bacteria you need for good health.

Vegetable oil will supply the fat you need for good body chemistry and to aid the absorption of fat-soluble vitamins.

Make sure that your diet contains some of all types of natural foods—with only a small amount of animal fat—and you'll get all the essential food elements you need to combat disease and delay the aging process. *Remember that food provides the most effective remedy we have for the aging process and all its effects.*

How to Relieve the Symptoms of Aging with Improved Circulation

Jasper R. complained of weakness and sluggishness that made him feel much older than his 54 years. "I eat good, Doc," he said, "and I even take vitamins. But I still feel old and decrepit."

It didn't take me long to figure out what Jasper's trouble was. Day after day of sitting at his desk had allowed circulatory stagnation, so that his tissue cells were not receiving adequate oxygen and nourishment. I recommended three simple measures that could be used right in his office. The benefits were evident almost immediately. "I not only feel better," he said, "I can now *think* better. I'm going to recommend that all my office workers do the same thing you have recommended for me."

Here's the three-step program I recommended for Jasper:

Step 1: pump blood with muscles

Walk briskly to the corner and back, swinging your arms in the process. Contraction of muscles all over your body will activate muscular pumps that will replace stagnant blood with a fresh flow of rich arterial blood. This will transport nutrients to aged, worn, and fatigued tissue cells so that they may be rejuvenated or replaced with new cells. Remember that the cells of your body are constantly being replaced.

Step 2: breathe to aid circulation

Immediately after completing the walk, sit down in front of a desk, place both hands palms-down on the desk top, and inhale deeply while pressing lightly against the desk top with your hands. Lift your chest as high as you can with each breath. Take as many deep breaths as necessary to satisfy your need for oxygen. Stop when you begin to feel a little dizzy.

The action of your diaphragm and certain chest muscles in this breathing exercise will pull blood up through the big veins leading to your heart, thus increasing the amount of blood being pumped through your lungs. This will increase the amount of life-giving oxygen in your blood.

Step 3: relieve brain fatigue with a slant board

Lie down on a slant board, with your feet anchored at the high end of the board. About 12 inches of elevation should be adequate. The slightly upside-down position will relieve compression on your spine, restore organs to their proper position, and increase the flow of blood to your brain. A few minutes on a slant board each day will revitalize your mind and body by reversing the effects of gravity. The forgetfulness and poor memory of a fatigued and oxygen-starved brain will disappear as if by magic.

How to stimulate your circulation with a contrast bath

Bathing the skin first in hot water and then in cold water will stimulate the circulation of blood by drawing blood to the skin and then driving it deep into the tissues. The hot water will dilate or open the blood vessels, while the cold water will constrict or close them. This has a beneficial pumping effect that will flush out your body and speed replacement of worn-out tissue cells.

Remember, however, that the older you become the more sluggish your circulation becomes. This means that your heart and blood vessels may be slow reacting to sudden changes in temperature. So try to avoid bathing in water so cold that a chill occurs. Be guided by comfort. Expose your body to cold water gradually by slowly turning the water from hot to cold. This can be done most conveniently in a shower.

How to Rebuild Your Body with Sleep

Most of the repair and restoration of your body occurs during the night when you sleep. Energy stores are replenished and tissues are repaired. And while all this is going on, a drop in blood pressure, heart rate, and respiration gives your vital organs a much needed rest. Without adequate sleep, wear and tear will exceed repair, and chronic fatigue will speed the aging process. So no matter what you do during the day to improve your health and relieve the symptoms of aging, you should make sure that you get several hours of sound sleep each night. The first four hours of sleep are the deepest and therefore the most important.

There are many people who get along fine with only four or five hours of sleep each night. There is, however, some evidence to indicate that *persons who average seven to eight hours of sleep each night have the longest life expectancy.*

Sleep is a potent remedy!

There's no doubt that sleep is a great healer. Yet, millions of people fail to get adequate sleep each night. Most of them feel tired, nervous, run down, and very often depressed. A disc jockey, for example, who also owned a gift shop, went through several extensive medical checkups trying to find the cause of a "nervous tremor" and a variety of vague aches and pains before he discovered that all he needed was a little extra sleep. "I still have my radio program," he reported later, "and I still work some in my gift shop. But I take naps during the day—and I feel fine." Had the hard-working disc jockey continued to skimp on sleep, the wear and tear on his body would have eventually led to the development of aging disease.

Six simple remedies for insomnia

Use one or more of these remedies for insomnia and you'll sleep like a baby. Best of all, many of those symptoms of premature aging will disappear.

Regular sleeping hours. Go to bed at the same time each night. Regular sleeping hours will condition your nervous system so that you will be able to fall asleep as a matter of habit.

A comfortable bedroom. Make sure that the environment of your bedroom is comfortable—free from noise, drafts, lights, and other disturbing influences.

Avoid stimulating drinks. Do not drink coffee, tea, cola, or cocoa with your evening meals. These beverages contain nervous-system stimulants that may keep you awake.

Don't overload your stomach. A light bedtime snack will help induce sleep by drawing blood from your brain to your stomach. An overloaded stomach, however, will put your nerves on edge and keep you awake. Salty foods may also keep you awake by stimulating your adrenal glands and raising your blood pressure.

Use nature's tranquilizers. Calcium is a natural tranquilizer. If you're a "light sleeper" and your nerves keep you awake, take a little calcium, or drink a glass of warm milk sweetened with a spoonful of honey. A little brewer's yeast powder added to the milk will enrich it with nerve-calming B vitamins.

Magnesium is also a natural tranquilizer. Health food stores sell tablets containing balanced amounts of calcium and magnesium. Prolonged use of only calcium may actually result in a deficiency in magnesium.

Relax with a warm bath. A warm bath will relax muscles at bedtime. When you do go to bed, concentrate on relaxing so completely that your muscles sag lifelessly. If you make sure that the muscles of your face are relaxed, chances are the rest of your muscles will also be relaxed. Erase unsolved problems from your mind. Think about the things you enjoy doing. If you succeed in relaxing your mind as well as your muscles, you won't have any trouble falling asleep.

Note: For more information on sleeping better and building youthful health for a long life, refer to my book *Secrets of Naturally Youthful Health and Vitality* (Parker Publishing Company, West Nyack, New York 10994).

Summary

1. Premature aging and disease, caused by bad living habits, cut the average person's life span in half.
2. Good nutrition combined with measures designed to stimulate the circulation of blood will delay the aging process and aid the healing powers of the body.
3. Vitamin C prevents sagging of tissues by building strong tissue cells and by strengthening the connective tissue that holds the cells together.
4. Vitamin E combats the aging process by preventing oxidation of tissues and fatty acids.
5. Without adequate calcium, tissue cells grow old prematurely because of an inability to exchange wastes for nutrients.
6. *All* of the known vitamins and minerals, supplied by fresh, *natural* foods, are essential to good health and a long life.
7. Depend upon fruits and vegetables for your carbohydrate, and stay away from refined foods.
8. Walking, deep breathing, use of a slant board, and proper use of water tonics will delay the aging process by aiding the circulation of blood.
9. Adequate sleep each night is essential for recovery and repair of worn and aging tissue cells.
10. A little honey and brewer's yeast mixed into a glass of warm milk will give you a sleep-producing drink that's rich in calcium and B vitamins.

14

How to Boost Your Sex Life and Ease the Strain of the Menopause and the Male Climacteric

Menopause for the female usually begins between the ages of 45 to 50. For some women, the menopause is the beginning of a new and better way of life, with more sexual freedom and no monthly inconvenience or discomfort. For others, it means nervousness and worry about "middle age madness." Actually, menopause is a normal, natural process, and there is no reason why every woman cannot make the change with little or no trouble. And there should be no marked decline in sexual appetite. Many women experience an *increase* in sexual desire when they are freed from the fear of pregnancy.

Most of the problems of menopause are created by ignorance and intolerance. A woman who believes that the "change of life" means an end to her sex life, for example, may withdraw from her husband and allow her physical condition to deteriorate. This may lead to emotional problems caused by the rejection of her husband who no longer finds her physically attractive. In this roundabout way, her sexual activities do come to an end, but not because of the effects of the menopause.

It appears that some men also experience a sort of menopause, a "male climacteric," that brings nervous and sexual problems. Many doctors believe that this change is simply *emotional difficulty* in coping with the realities of life. A middle-aged man, for example, who finds his sexual powers waning, or who must face the realization that his life-long ambitions will never be fulfilled, may be filled with such emotional despair that he loses every bit of the confidence and ambition he once had. There is some evidence, however, to indicate that *deterioration of glands* that produce male sex hormones may result in declining sexual ability along with physical and emotional symptoms.

Note: Any man over forty who has sexual problems should be checked for diabetes before assuming that he is simply undergoing a change of life. One man who was a heavy sugar eater reported that his sexual powers were restored after going on a sugar-free diet to control a mild case of diabetes.

Help for Men and Women in the Grip of Menopause

There are many things that a man or woman can do to ease the problems that occur during the "change of life." Nutritional supplements, for example, will soothe nerves, restore vigor, and improve physical appearance. When the nerves become jangled, or when sexual powers start fading, special attention to both your state of mind and your physical condition can mean the difference between success and failure in maintaining a happy marriage. Personal hygiene, physical grooming, provocative dress, and a few kind or sympathetic words can do wonders in giving your marriage a boost. Mental attitude alone is so important that every man or woman who is struggling with change-of-life problems would benefit from the moral support offered by an understanding mate.

Not every woman has trouble with the menopause. In many cases, menstruation ceases without any symptoms whatsoever. Others experience the expected hot flashes, periods of depression, irritability, and other symptoms. Kathleen J., for example, was only 44 when she first began to experience menopausal difficulties. Her doctors advised against the use of estrogen hormones because of a history of breast and uterine cancer in her family background. "I have to do something," she pleaded, "or my husband is going to leave me. I'm getting so nervous and irritable that I can't stand myself—and I'm getting old and ugly!"

Actually, Kathleen wasn't a bit ugly, and she certainly wasn't old. A few simple remedies and suggestions eased her nerves and boosted her vitality. "I'm still having an occasional hot flash," she reported, "but otherwise I'm getting along fine—and my sex life is better than ever."

Hints for the Menopausal Woman

Keep yourself as attractive as possible. Most women find that if they make an effort to remain as attractive and as appealing as possible, their own desires are stimulated by the interest of their husband. In this way, they avoid the vicious cycle that begins when physical deterioration and lack of love begin to feed one another.

Improve your physical appearance by walking off tension

When nervousness, anxiety, and irritability begin to build, a small amount of exercise will often relieve the tension. A walk around the block, a bicycle trip, or any physical activity that warms your muscles and produces a mild physical fatigue will relax nerves. Your physical appearance will also benefit from improved muscle tone and better circulation. *Exercise is a great tranquilizer, and it has no harmful side effects.*

Use a natural calcium tranquilizer

Calcium absorption is often poor after menopause. It's well known that a calcium deficiency can cause a great variety of nervous symptoms (as well as brittle bones). So it might be a good idea to take a supplement containing calcium (and magnesium) when you begin to feel a little jumpy.

Note: Blood calcium also drops during menstruation, causing cramps and menstrual tension. Adelle Davis says that if adequate calcium is obtained and efficiently absorbed, both premenstrual tension and menstrual cramps can be prevented. She recommends one or two calcium tablets every hour for relief from cramps. Vitamin B complex is also a good nerve tonic.

You'll find plenty of hints on how to get immediate relief from tension if you'll go back and read Chapter 3.

Sponge away hot flashes

When hot flashes are prolonged and uncomfortable, sponging with alcohol or cold water will provide relief by constricting dilated blood vessels. Vitamin B complex and Vitamin E will help normalize circulation.

Quick relief for fatigue and other symptoms

Fatigue is a common menopausal complaint. The wet-sheet rub, described in Chapter 12, will pep you up in an emergency. A change in the daily routine will sometimes relieve fatigue caused by "nerves." A high-protein diet with Vitamin C will help keep energy levels high.

Many other complaints of menopause, such as insomnia, headache, and a variety of aches and pains will respond to various home remedies. Warm baths, for example, can be used to relax tense nerves. Cool baths will wake up tired nerves, and so on. Whatever your complaint, you can find an effective home remedy in one of the chapters of this book.

A variety of fresh, natural foods, along with basic natural food supplements containing the essential vitamins and minerals, will help you through the menopause. Calcium, B complex, and Vitamin E are probably most important, and these should be taken in fairly large amounts. About 300 units of Vitamin E daily, for example, are usually recommended. One famous nutritionist says that hot flashes, night sweats, leg cramps, irritability, nervousness, and mental depression can usually be overcome in a single day by giving adequate calcium.

In addition to taking vitamin and mineral supplements, use bone meal, wheat germ, and brewer's yeast as additives in preparing your foods. Bone meal, for example, can be added to homemade bread. Brewer's yeast powder can be sprinkled over foods or mixed in beverages. Wheat germ can be mixed with cereals, and so on.

Note: Pre-menstrual tension will often respond to the same measures recommended for menopausal complaints. Regular use of these measures *before* menopause begins will often delay the menopause and contribute to a trouble-free change. Anything you can do to improve your health will give you the strength and the body chemistry you need to withstand the hormone changes of middle age.

Relief for the Aging Vagina

Senile vaginitis is a common problem among women after menopause. In this condition, the membrane lining the vagina becomes thin, dry, and sensitive, and is easily torn. As a result, sexual intercourse may be painful or irritating. Special vaginal creams containing estrogenic hormones will do wonders in relieving this condition. Foods containing Vitamin E should also help.

Note: If you have ever had cancer, you should not take estrogen orally or by injection since it might activate dormant cancer cells.

How to clean an irritated vagina

Excessive douching should be avoided when there are no vaginal complaints. When douching must be used often, in vaginitis or because of a discharge, use two quarts of water that contains one teaspoonful of lactic acid or three tablespoons of white vinegar. This will help maintain the normal acid environment of the vagina.

In simple vaginitis, glycogen tablets are often inserted into the vagina (following a lactic acid douche) so that the action of the bacteria on the glycogen will *produce* lactic acid. (Infection occurs much more readily in an alkaline vagina than in an acid vagina.)

In a healthy woman, the normal secretions of the vagina will keep it clean and acid. When it's necessary to use an occasional cleansing douche, two teaspoons of salt in two quarts of water will suffice.

When you insert a douche tip into your vagina, seal it off with your hand so that the water will fill the vagina and stretch out the folds in the vaginal walls. Then release the water and repeat the irrigation. Do this until you have used two quarts of water.

How to Reverse the Male Change of Life

Although there is still some controversy about whether men experience a "change of life" that's similar to the female menopause, there is no doubt that many men do experience a decline in mental, physical, and sexual abilities after middle age. And in many cases, they become as irritable, depressed, and emotionally unstable as a woman having a difficult menopause. Some nutritionists believe that these changes do not occur in men who live and eat properly. Like many other diseases that afflict the aging male, the male climacteric may be a degenerative process that is not a normal part of the aging process. If this is the case, it can be prevented or relieved by healthful living.

When a middle-aged man's problems are emotional in origin, the tender, reassuring care of a loving wife is the best remedy. One of my patients, Leroy B., confessed to me that he had once contemplated suicide when his business failed and his sexual powers diminished. "The only thing that saved me," he said, "was my wife. She stood behind me until I could get started again, and she was constantly reassuring me. We still don't make love as often as we used to, but we've both learned that quality is better than quantity."

Home Care for Prostate Troubles

Most men begin to have a little prostate trouble after 50 years of age. The gland usually enlarges and becomes inflamed or interferes with the passage of urine. Inability to empty the bladder completely, because of partial obstruction by a swollen prostate, causes frequent urination, especially during the night. "I have to get up half a dozen times every night to go to the bathroom and dribble," complained Wilbur E., a 60-year-old retired air force colonel. "And the sleep I'm losing is ruining my health. Prostate massages do not seem to help."

Wilbur's prostate gland was so large that he could empty only a small portion of a full bladder. Just imagine how a dam holds back water except for the overflow and you can understand how an enlarged prostate gland can make it difficult to empty the bladder.

Backache, leg ache, fever, pain during a sexual climax, persistent erection of the penis, trouble emptying the bowels, and other symptoms can result from prostate trouble.

Wilbur E. followed the simple remedies I've outlined here for prostate trouble and reported considerable relief. "I don't have to get up as often at night," he said, "so I'm sleeping a lot better and feeling *much* better. I no longer have any pain when I make love, which makes things better for both me and my wife."

How to examine the prostate gland

In checking for an enlarged prostate gland, the examiner inserts a lubricated, rubber-gloved finger into the rectum. The gland can be felt on the front side of the rectum a few inches inside the rectal opening. It should be smooth, firm, and about the size of a walnut. If it is large, lumpy, hard, spongy, or sensitive, it may be diseased, swollen, or inflamed.

Note: When there is a prostate infection, separate urine specimens taken at the beginning and at the end of urination will usually be cloudy. Just collect a small amount of urine in a couple of clean glasses. Then hold the glasses up to the light and look for cloudiness.

How to relieve prostate congestion with a sitz bath

Daily hot sitz baths will often relieve the symptoms of prostate trouble by stimulating the flow of blood. Just sit in about four inches of water—112 degrees or less—for about 20 minutes.

The bladder can sometimes be emptied more completely by urinating while sitting in a tub of hot water. This may be a little messy, but it beats getting up at all hours of the night. Besides, it's important that you empty your bladder as completely as possible every day. Urine that remains in the bladder too long will become stagnant and inflame the sensitive lining of the bladder, and this can lead to infection or cystitis.

How to ease the sitting syndrome

Traveling or sitting for a long time, especially during a bumpy ride, can inflame a sensitive prostate. One man, for example, experienced complete relief from chronic prostate trouble when he gave up his job driving a road tractor.

Cold or dampness may also trigger prostate trouble. Be careful to avoid sitting on frozen ground, cold metal, and other chilling surfaces. When a chill does seem to inflame the prostate, apply hot, moist towels to your crotch or take a hot sitz bath.

Special vitamins and minerals for the prostate gland

Vitamin F in tablet form has been used successfully in the treatment of some types of prostate trouble. Vegetable oil contains Vitamin F, but it may not be rich enough for immediate results.

It has been reported that *raw pumpkin seeds* contain hormones (as well as Vitamin F and Vitamin E) that aid the function of the prostate gland.

The amino acids *glycine, alanine,* and *glutamic acid,* which can be found in any protein-rich food (brewer's yeast, milk, beef, soybeans, liver, and so on), have been found to be beneficial in relieving prostate trouble.

Zinc and magnesium are also believed to aid recovery from prostate trouble. (The fluid secreted by the prostate gland contains large concentrations of magnesium and zinc!) Wheat germ, beef liver, oysters, nuts, seeds, and whole grains are good sources of magnesium and zinc. Dolomite, a mineral mined from the earth, contains a large amount of magnesium. Oysters are especially rich in zinc, which may account for the tag they have received as a sex stimulant. Casanova claimed that he ate more than 100 oysters daily!

How to Restore Sexual Powers

Although sexual desire may decrease in men after 50 years of age, there isn't any reason why an "old" man or an "aging" woman cannot continue to enjoy sexual intercourse. Unfortunately, many men and women simply give up sex in their twilight years because "it's not a nice thing for old people to do." The concept of the "dirty old man" has been encouraged by an attitude that has persisted from a puritanical age. This attitude was expressed perfectly by Sam Levinson when he told of his childhood discovery of the origin of babies. "When I first found out babies were born," he said with tongue in cheek, "I couldn't believe it! To think that my mother and father would do such a thing . . . . My father—maybe, but my mother—never!"

Age should be no barrier to continued sexual activity as long as the desire is felt. It's true that many men and women seem to lose interest in sex after the age of 70, but there are many in their eighties who are still sexually active. One doctor tells of an 87-year-old man who complained that he was unable to have sexual relations more often than three times a week! This case may be unusual. But the point is this: *No matter how old you are, you should remain sexually active as long as you feel the desire.*

In many cases, an apparent lack of interest in sex can be reversed by a stimulating partner. Many "impotent" men, for example, have been revived by a change in the attitude of a wife or by the attention of a young, aggressive woman. So don't just assume that age always means an end to the pleasures of sex.

Keep your body as attractive as possible; stay healthy and vigorous by eating natural foods; live fully; and show an interest in your mate. You may find that you're not as old as you thought you were.

How to Use Vitamin E for Sexual Rejuvenation

Food supplements that supply *all* the basic vitamins and minerals will be helpful in maintaining youthful health and vigor. Vitamin E may be especially helpful. There is mounting evidence, for example, to indicate that concentrated, natural Vitamin E in capsule form does indeed boost sexual vigor. Wheat germ oil is one of the best food sources of Vitamin E, and it's great for maintaining health. But for illness and sexual problems, you need much more Vitamin E than you can get from food.

The minimum daily requirement for Vitamin E is given as 30 International Units. The average American diet, which is made up largely of refined and processed foods, supplies less than 12 units, which is obviously not enough. A couple of hundred units a day will be needed for a real boost, which means that the vitamin must be taken in capsule form. You should, of course, eat plenty of wheat germ, seeds, nuts, green leafy vegetables, whole grain products, and other natural foods containing Vitamin E. But when menopause or change-of-life problems begin, you need all the extra Vitamin E you can get.

A menopausal couple who rarely had sexual intercourse both started taking several hundred units of Vitamin E daily on the advice of their physician. In a matter of weeks, both began to experience greater vigor and endurance and an increasing desire for sexual activity. For the first time during their marriage, the husband was able to last long enough to satisfy his wife. "It's like being married for the first time," she said. "We're reading marriage manuals like newlyweds—and it's wonderful." Both appeared to be happy, energetic, and more youthful.

Laboratory tests have shown that the aging process can actually be slowed or reversed with adequate amounts of Vitamin E. Its effects in improving the circulation of blood and increasing the oxygen-carrying capacity of the blood is bound to increase sexual vigor by improving the vital functions of the body. *Continued sexual activity in itself is a stimulating tonic that will delay the aging process.* The physical performance of the sexual act is good exercise!

How to take Vitamin E

Most natural Vitamin E is in oil form. If you cannot tolerate oil, you can buy a special water-soluble Vitamin E.

Begin with 100 units a day and gradually increase the amount from day to day. Too large a dose to begin with may cause a temporary rise in blood pressure. Women can work up to 400 units a day; men, up to about 600 units a day. Take the vitamin three times daily, about 15 minutes before meals so that it will be more readily absorbed into your system.

Iron will interfere with the absorption of Vitamin E. So if you take iron supplements, wait 12 hours before taking Vitamin E. Mineral oil will wash Vitamin E right out of your intestinal tract, along with other oil-soluble vitamins. (It's all right to inject mineral oil into your rectum for its lubricating effects, but you should be cautious about taking it orally.)

If you depend upon wheat germ or wheat germ oil for Vitamin E, remember that they lose Vitamin E when they become rancid. Keep them sealed and refrigerated when they aren't being used. Remember, however, that one teaspoonful of wheat germ oil contains only about 10 units of Vitamin E. You can use wheat germ oil in cooking and on salads, or you may take it from a spoon, but you may not be able to depend upon it for the amount of Vitamin E you need for relief from menopausal symptoms.

Summary

1. Good health and a healthy attitude can mean a new and better life for women who have gone through the menopause.
2. The best remedy for a man who is experiencing change-of-life symptoms is a loving, understanding wife.
3. Calcium with magnesium is a natural tranquilizer that will relieve many pre-menstrual and menopausal symptoms.
4. Senile vaginitis will respond quickly to vaginal creams that contain estrogenic hormones.
5. Douche water containing a small amount of lactic acid or white vinegar will maintain the normal acid environment of the vagina.
6. Dribbling or difficulty in emptying the male bladder can often be relieved by sitting in hot water to relieve prostatic congestion.
7. Vitamin F, zinc, magnesium, and certain amino acids have been found to be beneficial in relieving prostate trouble.
8. Continued sexual activity throughout one's life is a stimulating tonic that will delay the aging process.
9. Concentrated, natural Vitamin E supplements will boost sexual vigor in both men and women.
10. A variety of fresh, natural foods, with emphasis on wheat germ, seeds, nuts, whole grains, and green leafy vegetables, will build resistance against aging and sexual deterioration.

15

Miscellaneous Naturomatic Remedies for a Variety of Injuries and Ailments

If you didn't find your particular ailment discussed in other chapters of this book, you may find it in this chapter—that is, if it's something you can handle at home. There are many serious diseases that must be treated only under the supervision of a physician. Fortunately, most of the ailments we suffer from *can* be helped at home. No matter how healthy we think we are, *all* of us will eventually suffer from some of the common ailments. Right now, for example, you might be suffering from backache, varicose veins, tendonitis, or any one of the multitude of ailments that plague the average person. Even if you feel fine, you know that tomorrow may bring strains, sprains, constipation, aching feet, a sore throat, a cold, or some other common or uncommon ailment. So be sure to keep this book handy for use as a guide every time a new ailment crops up. The natural remedies you find on every page of this book will build your health as well as relieve your symptoms.

How to Heal Cystitis or Bladder Infection

Inflammation of the bladder is very common in women, mainly because of a short urinary tube (urethra) that allows the entrance of germs. (Women should always clean the anal area by wiping from front to back, using each piece of tissue only once. Otherwise, germs from the rectum may be pushed toward the vaginal area where they enter the urethra.)

Frequent urination accompanied by pain and a burning sensation may be the first symptoms of cystitis, followed by cloudy or bloody urine. This usually means that the lining of the bladder and the urinary tube are raw and inflamed. The acid urine burns the sensitive membranes, causing erosion and bleeding that leads to even more severe infection.

At the first sign of an inflamed or infected bladder, begin drinking a glass of water or fruit juice every 20 to 30 minutes. The more liquids you drink the better, since this will flush out your bladder and dilute your urine so that it will be less irritating. Fruit and vegetable juices will alkalize your urine and reduce the pain and burning—and the damage—caused by normally acid urine.

If you don't have high blood pressure or kidney trouble, you can put a little baking soda in your drinking water or in lemonade. This will help alkalize your urine when pain and burning are severe. Remember, however, that baking soda will also neutralize stomach acid, and if used excessively will result in illness caused by alkalosis.

A low-protein diet consisting mainly of fresh fruits and vegetables, with very little meat, bread, milk, or cereal, will help keep your urine alkaline until your bladder heals.

A hot sitz bath or a hot fomentation applied over the pubic area will relieve cramping discomfort.

How to Cope with Rectocele

Women who have given birth to children often have such a weak vaginal wall that the rectum tends to bulge forward into the vagina, making it difficult to empty the bowels. If you start having such trouble, sit in a flexed posture with your feet on a low stool when you use the toilet. Or simply squat down, as the Japanese do, to empty your bowels. This will force the bowel to empty toward the back rather than toward the front where the vagina is located.

How to Handle Frostbite

Prolonged exposure of the fingers, toes, nose, ears, and other prominent parts of the body to freezing temperatures may result in frostbite or frozen tissue. The skin first becomes white and then changes to a dark red color with complete loss of sensation. In a severe case, the skin actually turns black.

You should *never* rub frozen flesh with snow. Instead, heat water to a temperature between 100 and 104 degrees and pour it over the frozen part. It's very important to make sure that the temperature of the water does not go above or below these temperatures, since damage to the tissues occurs if thawing is too fast or too slow. Too much heat, for example, can result in gangrene. When warm water is not available, cover the frozen limb with a blanket and let it thaw gradually. Do not use a heating pad or a heat lamp—and do not rub the frozen tissue. Hot drinks will aid warming. An alcoholic drink will relieve pain and speed recovery by dilating blood vessels.

How to Handle Heat Illness

Heat stroke: When heat stroke occurs from prolonged exposure to hot air or the sun's rays, *perspiration ceases, the skin becomes red, hot, and dry,* and the body temperature begins to rise. Unconsciousness may also occur. It's extremely important to cool the victim immediately. If body temperature goes above 105 degrees, damage to the nervous system may occur, resulting in death or disability.

Immersion in a tub of water and giving an underwater massage to the arms and legs is the best way to cool the body and reduce temperature. The application of cold towels while a fan is blowing over the body will also provide effective cooling. The cooling should be discontinued when the rectal temperature reaches 103 degrees Fahrenheit; otherwise, the body temperature may drop too low and lead to shock.

Whatever cooling method you use, keep the head elevated. Remember: "When the face is red, elevate the head."

Heat exhaustion: When heat exhaustion occurs, the victim may suddenly experience weakness, nausea, and headache, and he may even faint. But throughout it all, he'll be *sweating profusely,* and there'll be little or no change in body temperature. The skin will be cold and clammy rather than hot and dry as in heat stroke. Let the victim lie down—with his head low—in a cool spot and give him mildly-salted fluids. One teaspoonful of salt in a quart of water will do. Keep an eye on him for signs of heat stroke.

How to Stop Nausea

When you are nauseated for no apparent reason, a day-long fast, followed by a day of fruit juices and soups before beginning again with solid foods, will give your stomach a chance to clean itself out. Sucking on ice chips during the fast may help.

How to Ease Gas Pains

When you are troubled with gas pains in your lower abdomen, a simple enema made up of one quart of water that contains two teaspoons of oil of peppermint may bring relief (see Chapter 9). Warm water may be best, but make sure that it's not above 112 degrees. Retain the water for about five minutes before releasing it.

You can get rid of gas pockets in your colon by getting down on your knees and elbows so that your hips will be higher than your abdomen. The gas will rise to the rectum so that it can be expelled.

Gas pains in the stomach, which are relieved by belching, are often caused by swallowing air, especially while chewing gum. Taking soda or an alkalizer to relieve such pain may only cause *more* gas when the alkali reacts with the stomach acid. Drinking a carbonated beverage will sometimes bring up stomach air by causing belching.

How to Stop Hiccups

A hiccup is a spasm of the diaphragm, the big, flat muscle that separates the chest cavity from the abdominal cavity. Most hiccups do not last very long, but they do occasionally last long enough to be aggravating.

Breathing into a paper bag to build up the amount of carbon dioxide in the blood is often effective in stopping hiccups. Deep breathing sometimes helps. Drinking a full glass of water without stopping, pulling on the tongue, putting pressure on the eyeballs, swallowing dry bread or crushed ice, placing an ice bag on the pit of the stomach, or putting light, fingertip pressure on the nerves and blood vessels on each side of the neck for about a minute will sometimes stop hiccups. Enemas and laxatives are sometimes prescribed to clean out the intestinal tract.

When hiccups persist and nothing seems to help, they may be the result of organic disease or a tumor.

If you have hiccups frequently, don't overeat, and avoid hot or spicy foods. Most of us have experienced hiccups after eating a big meal. This is usually caused by pressure on nerves that supply both the stomach and the diaphragm.

What to Do About Fever Blisters

Just about everyone has seen a fever blister. It's a small group of blisters, usually on the lip, that develops following an illness, stomach trouble, exposure to the sun, or some other disturbance that seems to weaken the body. The blisters are caused by a herpes simplex virus that lies dormant in the body until it is activated by stress or lowered resistance. Once the blisters develop, they usually run a course of seven to ten days and then dry up without leaving a scar.

If you have fever blisters frequently, and you know what it is that triggers them, you may be able to prevent them by taking a few thousand milligrams of Vitamin C daily for a couple of days *before* the blisters develop. Otherwise, the only sure remedy in some cases is to condition your body so that it will be less susceptible to the virus. If you get fever blisters after exercising or sunbathing, for example, it usually means that you simply aren't accustomed to these activities. The only way to avoid recurrence of the blisters is to gradually condition your body by exercising more and sunbathing more, until you become so accustomed to them that they do not put stress on your body's recovery powers.

I have exercised most of my life. As long as I exercise regularly, I can do so without any ill effects. But when I quit exercising for several weeks for some reason, a little unaccustomed exercise almost invariably causes a fever blister. Rather than suffer one of these blisters every time I exert myself physically, I would much prefer the inconvenience of a little regular exercise.

Emotional stress causes fever blisters in some people.

Note: The virus in a fresh fever blister may be contagious. So it might be a good idea to avoid direct, intimate contact with your wife or girl friend while the blisters are on your body. My wife contracted her first fever blister from me during the early days of our marriage, and she has had them regularly ever since.

Hints on the Care of Shingles

The blisters that occur in shingles are very much like those seen in fever blisters. They are, in fact, caused by a virus called herpes zoster that is similar to the herpes simplex virus that causes fever blisters. Most of the time, shingles follow the course of a nerve around the chest or abdomen, although they can occur anywhere on the body. Like fever blisters, they usually run a course and then disappear. Scarring occurs, however, and the affected nerve may cause pain long after the skin has healed.

There is no specific treatment for shingles, but a moist cold pack or hot pack might help relieve the burning, stabbing pain. Heavy doses of Vitamin B Complex (with B_{12}) may be helpful in speeding recovery. Painting the skin with collodion (available in drug stores), oatmeal water, or a cornstarch solution (see Chapter 11) might help relieve symptoms.

Don't worry about shingles being fatal if they encircle your body. This is an old wive's tale that has no basis in fact.

How to Treat Rosacea

This is a form of acne that reddens the nose and cheeks and sometimes causes the nose to enlarge. Rubbing the red areas with ice and washing the face frequently with soap and cold water will reduce the redness. Hot foods and drinks, spicy foods, and alcoholic beverages can aggravate rosacea by flushing the face with blood. Try to avoid extreme heat.

Use cold packs, cold water, or ice massage as often as possible to prevent enlargement of the blood vessels in your nose. Many people who suffer from rosacea are often suspected of being heavy drinkers—an unfair and false suspicion.

How to Eliminate Hives

Itching followed by the appearance of a crop of wheals or pink bumps is usually hives, which means that you have been exposed to something that has resulted in an allergic reaction. Most of the time, the hives will disappear in a few days or a few weeks.

Emotional stress can cause hives by triggering the release of histamine in tiny nerve endings in the skin. Food allergy, however, is the most common cause of allergic reactions in the skin. Many people are sensitive to certain seasonal fruits and vegetables, which accounts for the appearance of hives during certain months of every year. Shellfish, nuts, eggs, wheat, milk, pork, and onions are common year-round offenders.

A mild laxative, a short fast, and plenty of drinking water will speed recovery by cleaning out the bowels. Baths containing cooked cornstarch, oatmeal squeezings, or a little sodium bicarbonate will usually relieve itching. See Chapter 11 for guidance in preparing itch-relieving baths.

How to Restore Color to Gray Hair

Some nutritionists maintain that premature gray hair is the result of a vitamin deficiency. Folic acid, para-aminobenzoic acid, and pantothenic acid, for example, which are B vitamins, are believed to play a part in the prevention of gray hair. So many different food elements play a part in the maintenance of a healthy head of hair that you cannot afford to be deficient in *any* of the essential elements. If your hair lacks luster or color, or if it's breaking off or falling out, you might be able to restore it with concentrated natural food supplements.

Yogurt, liver, yeast, and wheat germ contain elements believed to be important in preserving normal hair color. "Persons who take five milligrams of folic acid and 300 milligrams of both para-aminobenzoic acid and pantothenic acid daily with some B vitamins from natural sources," says one famous nutritionist, "can usually prevent hair from graying and often restore its color."

Brewer's yeast is the richest natural source of B vitamins.

How to Erase Skin Wrinkles

If your skin is dry and wrinkled, rub your skin with vegetable oil, such as olive oil, and then scrape the oil off with a rubber spatula. This will soften and smooth your skin as well as clean pores and remove dead tissue cells.

Vegetable oil used as a dressing on green salads will supply the unsaturated fatty acids you need for a soft, healthy skin. Vitamins A and C will keep the cells of the skin strong and youthful and prevent sagging.

Remember that sunlight ages the skin, so don't try to maintain a dark tan.

Rubbing your skin with a handful of wet corn meal will "sand" the rough spots off your skin.

How to Ease the Swelling of a Black Eye

A cold steak applied to the eye is a time-honored remedy for a black eye. It's not the steak, however, that prevents discoloration and swelling—it's the *cold*. So rather than use an expensive steak, you may simply use an insulated ice bag or a cold pack. Apply the cold pack as soon after the injury as possible. Leave it on for about 15 minutes at a time—several times over a period of 12 hours or so.

How to Get a Cinder Out of Your Eye

When an irritating particle gets under an eyelid, follow this procedure: If the particle is under the bottom eyelid, have a member of your family pull the lid down (while you look up) and dab out the particle with a cotton bud or a wisp of tissue paper.

If the particle is under the upper eyelid, the lid must be rolled over a match stick (while you look down) to expose the particle, which may then be dabbed out. Pressing down just a little with the match stick will expose a greater portion of the inner surface of the lid.

Simply spreading the eyelids apart with the thumb and fore-finger of one hand, so that the lids are pulled away from the eyeball, may permit a flow of tears to wash the cinder to the corner of the eye where it may be dabbed out.

Dust in the eye can be washed out with salt water (one-half teaspoon of salt in a pint of water) applied with an eyedropper or an eye cup.

How to Clean Out Your Ears

A few drops of warm olive oil or glycerine in the ear will ease earache, soften plugs of ear wax, and float out insects and other particles. Warm water in a rubber ear syringe can then be used to wash out the loose material. Water should not be used very often, however, since it may contribute to the growth of ear fungus. Always tilt your head to one side to drain water out of the ear, and then dry the ear canal with a cotton bud or a Q-tip.

Applying heat to the ear with a hot water bottle or a heating pad will often relieve ear pain.

Note: Arthritis in a jaw joint often causes pain in the vicinity of the ear. If your jaw pops or grinds when you chew, or if missing teeth do not permit you to chew evenly, inflammation of a jaw joint can cause what appears to be an earache.

How to Strengthen a Ruptured Abdomen

A hernia occurs when a portion of the intestine pushes through a rupture in the abdominal wall. This can occur anywhere around the abdomen, but it occurs most often in the groin area. In men, the hernia usually bulges through the inguinal ring near the pubic bone, while in women it most often bulges through the femoral ring a little higher up in the groin. Fortunately, both of these rings are surrounded by muscles. This means that a hernia in its early stages can often be corrected by developing these muscles. The thicker the muscles are, for example, the smaller the femoral and inguinal rings. And if the muscles are sufficiently developed to fit snugly around the structures that normally pass through these rings, there won't be any room for the intestinal tract to bulge through.

A massive hernia must be repaired surgically, but a hernia in its early stages can often be controlled with exercise. One man, for example, who had some bulging in his groin was able to eliminate the bulging by developing his abdominal muscles. "The last time I saw my doctor," he said, "there was no visible evidence of the hernia. I've been doing the sit-up exercise you recommended, so it must have helped."

If your doctor tells you that you have an enlarged "ring" that makes you subject to hernia, you may be able to *prevent* the hernia by developing your abdominal muscles *before* the bulge appears.

Whether you have a hernia or not, do this exercise: Lie down on a slant board with your feet anchored at the high end of the board. Curl only your head and shoulders up from the board (12 or 15 times). Concentrate on contracting your abdominal muscles. Exhale during each contraction.

Note: A bulging hernia can often be reduced by using your fingers to manipulate the intestine back through the opening while you are lying relaxed on a slant board. A truss may then be used to close the opening.

Always exhale when you are lifting or straining so that internal pressure won't build up and push your intestine back through the opening. Taking a deep breath and holding it during a heavy exertion or while contracting the abdominal muscles is a common cause of hernia.

How to Reduce Nervous Tremors

Magnesium and Vitamin B_6 (pyridoxine) have been recommended for muscle twitching and shaking hands. Even palsy, or Parkinson's disease, will sometimes improve if an adequate diet is supplemented with magnesium, Vitamin B_6, and Vitamin B complex.

How to Wrap Stubbed Toes and Fingers

The next time you stub your toe and you're worried that it might be broken, you may simply tape the toe to the adjoining toe for support. The big toe, however, may be taped alone if some of the tape reaches over onto the top of the foot for additional support.

A special finger wrap. If you sprain a finger so badly that movement is painful, you can splint it with a special rigid bandage. Wrap the finger with a couple layers of one-inch gauze and then paint them with collodion. After the collodion drys, lay a large U-shaped hairpin over the finger and wrap it again with a couple more layers of gauze, followed by another coat of collodion. Keep applying gauze and collodion until the finger is covered with a sturdy, cast-like dressing.

Collodion is a plaster-like substance that can be purchased in any drug store.

How to Lose Excess Body Fat

When I advise my overweight patients on how to lose weight, I never give them a diet that requires them to count calories or measure food portions. It has been my experience that simply limiting food intake to fresh, *natural* foods will usually result in a loss of excess body fat. This means completely eliminating refined or processed foods, with absolutely nothing containing white sugar or white flour.

Recent research has revealed that a refined food is about *three times* more fattening than a natural food containing an equal number of calories. One of the reasons for this is that a refined carbohydrate is so rapidly absorbed into the blood stream that a sudden rise in blood sugar triggers an insulin reaction that immediately stores the sugar as fat. So much sugar may be removed from the blood that there is not enough left to meet the energy needs of the body, which explains why heavy sugar eaters are usually tired as well as fat. A natural carbohydrate, on the other hand, is absorbed and assimilated more slowly, requiring a metabolic process that burns calories while it feeds the body's energy machine. This means that you can get fatter—and have less energy—on a diet of white bread than on a diet of apples, even if both have the same number of calories.

If you'll concentrate on eating fresh fruits, vegetables, lean meat, fish, poultry, cottage cheese, skim milk, green salads, eggs, and whole grain products, your weight will eventually normalize. It's important, however, that you not use grease or oil in cooking. Bake or broil your meats. Eat frequent small meals rather than two or three large meals. Natural foods won't artificially stimulate your appetite, and you'll find that you'll be eating less and enjoying it more.

"I've had a weight problem for years," confessed Sherry W., a 39-year-old typist, "and I've been on plenty of diets. I usually end up starving myself to lose weight that I eventually gain back. Your natural foods diet is the first diet I have ever been able to stick with—and it really works!"

Sherry lost *all* of her excess body fat over a period of several months, and she never did suffer from hunger. "I now prepare all my food at home," she said, "so that my whole family can get the health benefits of natural foods."

If you have a stubborn weight problem, you may have to follow Sherry's example and fix your own meals in order to make sure that you get the type of food you need. It's difficult to lose weight when you eat in restaurants and sandwich shops.

Be as active as possible. Physical activity stimulates the body's metabolic processes so that there'll be less tendency for your body to store calories as fat. If you happen to be one of those unfortunate persons who has more fat cells than normal, you'll have to make a special effort to keep the cells from filling with fat. If you have ever been fat, chances are that your body has formed extra fat cells that will make it more difficult for you to maintain a lean body. If this is the case, a combination of exercise and diet will allow you to eat normally without gaining weight.

First Aid for Acid and Alkali Burns

The use of acids and alkalis in household cleaning chores sometimes results in painful burns. Donald A., for example, purchased a gallon of muriatic acid to clean a portion of a brick wall on his home. While he was diluting some of the acid with water, he accidentally knocked over the container of pure acid, splashing some on his feet. Quick thinking saved him from a serious burn. He immediately placed his foot under water running from a faucet. While he was doing that, his wife mixed a couple tablespoons of sodium bicarbonate into a quart of water. She soaked a dressing in the water, placed it over Donald's foot, and then poured the rest of the water over the dressing. Since sodium bicarbonate is an alkali, it neutralized the burning acid. Immersing an extremity in a solution of baking soda and water is a quick way to neutralize acid on the skin. Lime water or milk of magnesia can also be used in an emergency.

When lye, ammonia, or some other strong alkali is spilled on the skin, a fresh-water rinse followed by a dousing with water containing vinegar or lemon juice will prevent a bad burn. A dressing soaked in a mixture of vinegar and water can be applied over a deep burn.

First Aid for Spinal Fractures

A spinal fracture is not something that can be treated at home. How you handle it until the doctor arrives, however, can mean the difference between recovery and paralysis.

When a person falls and is unable to move his arms or his legs, *don't move him* unless it's absolutely necessary—at least not until an ambulance arrives.

If the injured person is unable to move his feet but can move his arms and fingers, his spine may be fractured somewhere below his neck. This means that he should be transported *face down* on a rigid stretcher.

If the victim is unable to move his feet *and* his fingers, his *neck* may be broken, which means that he should be transported *face up*.

Great care should be taken to make sure that the entire spine is kept straight and in proper alignment when lifting or turning the victim of a spinal fracture. This may require the assistance of several persons, one of whom must support the head in suspected neck fractures.

Nutritional Therapy for All Diseases

No matter what type of ailment you might be suffering from, you should make sure that your diet is rich in all the vitamins and minerals known to be essential for good health. A deficiency of any essential food element can play a part in the development of almost any type of disease. A wide variety of basic, natural foods will give your diet the balance it needs to combat disease. *No matter what type of pills or supplements you take, you still must eat the basic natural foods to be truly healthy.*

There are some less common natural foods that are especially concentrated in important vitamins and minerals. Wheat germ, brewer's yeast, fish liver oil, vegetable oil, bone meal, desiccated liver, rose hips, sunflower seeds, lecithin, and other popular items sold in health food stores can be added to your diet to boost your body's ability to overcome disease and infection.

Nutritional measures offer one of nature's most potent remedies for disease. The more you can learn about nutrition, the better.

Megavitamin therapy, in which large amounts of vitamins are used in the treatment of disease, is now being used by some doctors. Reportedly, many "incurable" diseases have been cured with massive doses of certain vitamins—with no harmful side effects. Glaucoma, for example, has responded to Vitamin C megavitamin therapy. Schizophrenia has been treated successfully with three grams of Vitamin B_3 (niacinamide) daily. So little is known about the effects of megavitamin therapy that almost any vitamin or combination of vitamins would be worth trying in the treatment of any disease that fails to respond to conventional treatment methods.

"Faulty cellular nutrition of one type or another may be a basic cause of most of the noninfective diseases—diseases that are at present poorly controlled by medical science,"* says Dr. Roger J. Williams, the nutritional biochemist who discovered the B vitamin pantothenic acid.

The role of nutrition in the treatment and prevention of disease has not yet been fully revealed. You can keep abreast of nutritional developments by reading such magazines as *Let's Live* and *Prevention,* which are available in health food stores.

Nutrition in a Nutshell. New York: Doubleday, 1962.

Summary

1. If you fail to find your ailment discussed in other chapters of this book, it might be covered in this chapter.
2. Use of the Index at the end of this book will help you locate the information you need to handle a great variety of common and not-so-common ailments.
3. The natural healing methods described in this book for the treatment of specific ailments will also build good health.
4. Every form of natural healing that can be used safely at home has been included in the various programs outlined in this book.
5. "Natural" is the key word of the future. As people become more knowledgeable about natural healing and self help, they will be rewarded with better health and a longer life.

Index